Breathing Again…
A Joyous Miracle

MY JOURNEY WITH
SCLERODERMA

Linda M. Edwards

GERE PUBLISHING

Breathing Again...A Joyous Miracle:
My Journey with Scleroderma

© 2016 Linda M. Edwards
ISBN 9780974399584
Gere Publishing

Contact: Linda Edwards
lmwe122@gmail.com

Printed in the United States of America

DEDICATION

I dedicate this book to all the people who are courageously handling their own challenge with positivity and determination.

Contents

Foreword

December 25, 2011

Dear Linda,

This past year has changed my perspective on life somewhat, as it undoubtedly has yours. I've learned the importance of family, the power of prayer, the meaning of courage, and the strength of positivity. But most importantly, I've learned that miracles do happen.

Over the last few years, you've wowed us with your hope, your fortitude, and your unwavering trust in God while you battled your disease.

By having that strength, you gave it to each of us. By believing in God's plan, you showed us how to trust him. By smiling through the pain, you helped us see all we had to smile about. Thank you.

In facing this hardship with the grace in which you have, you've reminded us who you are, and how integral you are to our family. And because God knew how much we needed you, he found you new lungs. He literally breathed new life into you when you needed it most. When we all needed it most.

We've all been given a second chance here—to stay close, love, and support each other, to appreciate the blessings we've been given, and to live each day like it's the prized miracle that it is. Thank you for showing us that miracles really do exist. You're living proof. LIVING proof.

All our love,

Katie and Clan

Acknowledgments

Thank you to my mother for your strength, presence, and solace throughout my ordeal, but especially during the time leading up to my surgery. Also to my brothers Tom and Joe and sisters Sue, Pat, and Nancy, who helped me tremendously throughout my journey for your loving support, sacrifice, patience and for being there when I needed you so much. I also appreciate your generous feedback as I wrote this book.

To my friend JoAnn, a special thanks for not only giving selflessly of your time but also for bringing me joy and laughter during some of the most difficult stages of my journey. As a language arts teacher, your contribution to this book was also invaluable.

To my niece Emily and nephew Dan who traveled by train to fill in at a critical time before my transplant, thank you so much for everything you did. Also thank you to my cousin Sandy for devoting three weeks of your time to care for me after the transplant. Your encouragement was so much appreciated and got me to the point of being independent again. You gave other family members much needed relief.

And to all the many other relatives, friends, and colleagues, my heartfelt thanks for being with me in my time of need through your visits, cards, phone calls, emails and prayers.

Thank you to the doctors, nurses and medical staff who took care of me...those mentioned in this book and those too numerous to acknowledge individually. A special thank you goes to Mary for the complementary holistic healing. My experience with energy healing was a life-changing experience as discussed in this book.

My thanks also go out to Claudia Gere, for bringing this book to life with your editing and publishing expertise. You have been a pleasure to work with including your professionalism.

Introduction

I decided to write a book about my experience with scleroderma and having a lung transplant caused by scleroderma. I thought it might be helpful to share my story to help others who might be going through a challenging medical condition or some other challenging situation. It was an amazing experience for me. I learned so much about myself and I learned the human body is incredibly strong. When you come so close to death and then come through it, you realize how precious life really is. Life is a gift and can be taken away when you least expect it. I don't take anything for granted anymore. Every minute of every day is appreciated even the simplest aspects of life.

1

Power of Positive Thinking

I've been living with scleroderma since I was thirty (1983) even though I didn't accept it until years later. I'm sixty-three now. I married at the age of "almost twenty one" (in 1973), way too young in retrospect, but I have to say I really wanted to explore life and was eager to leave my family nest at that time. My husband and I lived in Southern New Hampshire. I'm the type of person who likes to learn new things; I wasn't afraid of challenge. I started working at seventeen years old. I always strived to grow and better myself. I knew I was often times out of my comfort zone over the years, but I now know how important that is for personal growth and the later years in life. It has made me stronger. There are always new things to learn. The opportunities are there. You just have to be open to them.

I ended up not being able to have children due to issues with my fallopian tubes. I had one ectopic pregnancy, emergency surgery (lost a tube), and then a year later had micro tubal reconstruction surgery on the other tube, which turned out to be unsuccessful. Back in the late seventies, alternative procedures for becoming pregnant such as in vitro fertilization (IVF) were very costly and did not have a good success rate. My husband and I applied for adoption and were approved, but there was a waiting list to get on the waiting list. We were never given the chance to adopt, and it was a blow that I've had to work through my whole life, but I didn't let it defeat me.

I poured myself into my career and the friendships, socialization, and networking that comes with the working world, along with the friends and social life that came with my husband's advertising business. My husband and

I had a lot of friends and acquaintances (many with kids), and we held many social events at our home and were in turn invited to others' homes.

After eighteen years, though, our marriage failed. It doesn't matter why now. I just knew it was the right thing. I don't regret most of my married years. The experience is part of who I am. Not long after I was divorced and living on my own, still in Southern New Hampshire, at a local bookstore I came upon a book by Norman Vincent Peale. It was a thick book containing three complete books of his: *The Power of Positive Thinking*, *The Positive Principle Today*, and *Enthusiasm Makes the Difference*. This book of three literally changed my life and has stayed with me ever since.

It could not have come at a better time. Life throws you curveballs that you have to deal with as best you can. Being in the right state-of-mind is a tremendous asset. Peale's books helped me see life in a positive light. I believe our souls are going through experiences for a reason and according to God's Plan. We may not understand why, but I'm convinced there are no coincidences. The people we come in contact with, the experiences we encounter are all meant to happen for the growth of our soul. My faith in God was strengthened significantly after reading this book of three. It is much more fun to think positively than negatively. And it's so much more enjoyable to be around people who think positively.

This thought process changes your whole perspective on life. The glass is half full or half empty. I choose to see the glass half full. Eliminate the negative, accentuate the positive. I learned, "Experience is not what happens to you; it is what you do with what happens to you." This is a quote by Aldous Huxley. It stuck with me.

2

JANET

I do have twelve awesome nieces and nephews thanks to my siblings, and I love them all so much. I also have four nieces and nephews on my husband's side of the family who are very, very special. That helps. I'm a godmother five times and that means a lot to me.

While I was married, I was a Big Sister to a ten-year-old girl, Janet, who taught me a lot. She had an alcoholic mother, and the father was no longer in the picture in a different state. She was the oldest of four kids and had basically taken over as a mother of the younger ones. They lived in a project. Sometimes I would pick her up and she would come running out so happy to see me and have a piece of white bread rolled up in a ball. This was her after-school snack. She would show me in the project where the drug addicts were and areas to stay away from. No question about it, she taught me one side of the tracks, and I taught her another side. We had fun together.

I can remember it was around the time the song "We are the World," written by Lionel Richie and Michael Jackson, came out, and I had the single CD (it might have been a cassette tape now that I think about it), and we would play the song so loud and sing it so loud in my Audi with the sunroof open. We'd be laughing away. I took her to get haircuts periodically when she needed them. I would buy her clothes. Her mother was very appreciative since she really took no part in mothering her kids. She was drinking all the time. She cared enough to enroll Janet in the Big Brother Big Sister program so that says something.

Janet and I spent a good two years together. She went to certain events with me that I thought she would enjoy. My friends and my husband knew her and she knew

8

them. There were birthday parties, christenings, Halloweens, and so on. Then, sadly, she and her siblings had to go live with their father, I think in Tennessee. We wrote for a while but then lost touch. She was getting involved in a new environment and meeting new friends, which was a good thing. Years later after I had moved to Maryland and was in New Hampshire visiting my brother and his family, Janet and I bumped into each other at a restaurant. Was this a coincidence? I'll let you decide.

She was probably in her late teens. She was working at this restaurant. We both recognized each other. It was such a special moment. I was so happy to see her working. She looked good. She invited me to her apartment where she was living with her boyfriend. I was proud of her. I really do feel I made a difference in her life in some small way. She wasn't doing drugs or drinking. You could tell she didn't have a lot, but she seemed to be in the right frame of mind. She was a strong girl. I hope things are still going well for her.

3

SOMETHING IS BREWING

While living in Southern New Hampshire at thirty years old and still married, for ten years at this point (1983), my hands began to swell and the fingers started turning blue. My fingers would even get numb depending on how cold the temperature was. I also had a couple of tiny blue spots on my lips. Being concerned, my husband and I went to see a rheumatologist in the area. I remember the doctor saying he noticed beginning signs of scleroderma on my fingertips but it was nothing serious at this time. "Something is brew-

10

ing," he said, "We're going to have to wait it out."

We didn't really feel comfortable with that response so we went to Boston for a second opinion. I remember it was right before the Thanksgiving holiday. We were traveling to New Jersey for the holiday. I had some tests done prior to the trip including an angiogram to test for any blockage. There was no blockage. I was diagnosed with Lupus. I went all Thanksgiving weekend in New Jersey thinking I had Lupus, which didn't sound any better than scleroderma. I found out when I got home from New Jersey that the doctors had read the tests wrong. I did not have Lupus. I have Raynaud's phenomenon.

Raynaud's is a condition where your extremity vessels, those closest to the surface of your skin, are deteriorated. When your blood flows, it can't get to the extremity vessels since they are deteriorated thus causing discoloration and numbness. I didn't associate this with scleroderma. As far as I was told, I have Raynaud's. I have to be careful of the cold weather so my fingers don't get frostbite. Damp weather, stress, and caffeine can also be triggers of the swelling and discoloration. There is no treatment for Raynaud's except precautionary measures. Dress warm, wear mittens, manage stress, and limit caffeine are a few examples. Ok, so once I was aware of having this new condition, I managed to adjust.

Living in New Hampshire was not the mildest of climates. I loved to ski. I learned there are hand warmers in the ski stores that you put in your mittens while you ski. What a God send. Now you can get them everywhere. I was able to ski whenever I wanted.

I remember one night my husband and I went skiing. There was a beautiful moonlit sky that night, snowing, but not outrageously cold. Only problem was on one of the trips up the mountain on the chair lift, I dropped one of my mittens. It became an emergency. We were almost at the top of the mountain. Luckily there was a chalet. We immediately went inside. There was a fire in the fireplace, places to sit and relax. My mittenless hand was numb. You have to be careful not to go from cold to warmth too fast or it can cause a lot of discomfort. After I was settled, my husband went down the mountain and got a spare pair of mittens in the jeep and met me back up at the chalet. Problem solved. We continued to ski until closing. I was and still am so thankful to whoever invented those hand warmers. They are a life saver.

Getting into bed with my cold hands could be startling to a partner, but it didn't take long to warm up my hands with the body heat. Whenever I shook someone's hand I felt compelled to explain "cold hands, warm heart."

After my divorce in 1991, I was working to the max and adjusting to single life. I rented a condo a few towns away from where I had been living while married.

I discovered something new about my physical condition. I was having trouble swallowing when I ate or drank. It was as if my esophagus went into a spasm. I often times had to walk away from wherever I was and try to relax, concentrate on something positive, in hopes the spasm would subside. The food or liquid wouldn't come up or go down until the spasm went away (when it felt like it).

These episodes happened sporadically. They were unpredictable and very uncomfortable. One of the first episodes I had was on a British Columbia ski trip with a group of friends. We were at dinner in a restaurant when the spasm happened. I didn't remove myself from the table. I just stopped eating for a short period of time; long enough that the spasm went away, thankfully. But I remember it being odd and scary.

I tried to deal with it without anyone noticing. Another episode happened at a cousin's wedding in Connecticut. This spasm was bad. I got up and walked into the ladies' room. It took forever for the spasm to go away. It seemed that way anyway. My sister-in-law Michele followed me in to the ladies' room. The spasm just had to take its course. When it happened, I would say to people my esophagus is acting irresponsibly. It even happened on a one-on-one date once. It was uncomfortable for the both of us.

I attributed my esophagus problem to stress associated with getting a divorce and not being able to have children. This one particular time when my sister Sue and her daughter Katie came to visit me from Connecticut, I had another episode. They asked me, "How long has this been going on?"

I said, "Probably a couple of years." We initially laughed but we all knew it wasn't funny.

Sue said, "And you haven't gone to the doctor yet?"

It wasn't happening constantly, though, so I pressed on with work and life. I dealt with the spasms as scary as they were.

I loved meeting new people, traveling and having new life experiences. I worked a lot of hours. The training I was getting through work was interesting and helpful in both my work and personal life. Life is a give and take. You learn something new with each experience you have. Sometimes I make mistakes; don't we all. I came to realize it helps to take it with a grain of salt and know that you were meant to experience that mistake for personal growth. Everybody has their own feelings and thoughts that are valid. I learned that I needed to be able to communicate my thoughts and respect others' thoughts in the process leaving the emotion out of it as much as possible. It's not always easy to come to an agreement. You may have to agree to disagree, but at least you maintain mutual respect for each other. This skill plays a role at work, in families, and with friends.

One of the things that helped me learn interpersonal skills was in my job I had to lead proposal efforts as well as many other work efforts that involved a team of people (not always the same people) who didn't work directly for me. I had to learn how to motivate them to want to do the work and produce the results the company needed. I had to learn what makes each individual tick and work with each person to get the job done. The life experiences I was having helped greatly when I led a New Hampshire charity event called Tour de Cure for diabetes. At the time, my niece Katie had been diagnosed with juvenile diabetes, so there was extra meaning for me to be involved with this event. Subsequently, a nephew Mikey was also diagnosed with diabetes. They are both so brave.

There were all kinds of tasks that had to happen, and people that had to pull together to produce a successful event. I loved the challenge. I think humor and smiling are other good qualities to practice in life.

One day, my sister-in-law Anne who lived nearby came across an article she found, maybe in the newspaper, I can't remember now, but it was about scleroderma. She is a medical assistant. She mailed it to me with a note. She said "I think you have this." I didn't want to think about it. I was in denial. I didn't have time to deal with it.

4

CREST...NOT THE TOOTHPASTE

Eight years after being on my own in Southern New Hampshire, in 1999, feeling like I was in my prime, I moved to Silver Spring, Maryland with a job offer at a large company. They paid for my moving expenses. The company, itself, was in a prime area at the corner of Fourteenth and G Street in the District of Columbia.

I left my previous company after twenty-three years. These years are cherished, but I was emotionally ready to make a change and move on to something new. I was well prepared for this new opportunity.

I felt bad about leaving my brother and sister-in-law and their three kids who lived nearby. We were very close. But this was an opportunity I couldn't refuse. The rest of my family lived in Connecticut and Florida. I knew I could travel to see everyone. And I did. I'm the oldest of six. A few years back I came across a saying that has stuck with me. It said, "Pray to God but hammer away." It's a Spanish proverb. I always loved this saying. It put spring in my step. Little did I know the move to Maryland might have had more meaning than I realized. I was taking all the training and experience to a new level and now working in the city. I loved it. I loved life. I felt as good as I did when I was on vacation somewhere. I really did.

Initially, I have to admit I felt like a Beverly Hillbilly coming to the big city. Very fast paced. I got over the Hillbilly thing pretty quickly though. Not too long after I got to Maryland, I went to see a gastroenterologist about my esophagus situation. It had become a nuisance. I did learn from this GI specialist, after he performed an endoscopy, my esophagus muscle goes limp which causes food to not move down into the stomach and at the same time acid backs up from the stomach. The doctor told me I have esophagitis. He put me on an over-the-counter medication called Prilosec.

I didn't have much time to focus on my health. I was living in a new location and had a new job that I was enthusiastic about. I eventually had to get on a stronger prescription medication called Protonix. It does help lighten the impact on my daily life. But I continue to have unpredictable episodes to this day. Esophagitis is something that many people get so I didn't think too much about it. Raynaud's is also something that many people get, so I didn't think too much about this either. I didn't associate either one with scleroderma.

I should mention I had a cyst-like growth that was removed from my finger before my move to Maryland. It was a calcium deposit that formed in one of my fingers. I didn't think too much about this situation either, but it turned out to be significant. After my move to Maryland, I had two other calcium deposits surgically removed. I thought this was kind of strange. Was I producing too much calcium in my body, I thought to myself, "These cyst-like growths feel like pieces of coral you find in the ocean with sharp edges." They mainly develop in the hands and forearms. I have several other calcium deposits in my fingers and elbows but I tolerate them for now.

My primary care doctor (PCP) suggested I go see a rheumatologist. This was in 2000, about seven months after I moved to Maryland. He referred me to a doctor in Baltimore. This rheumatologist did blood tests and confirmed my diagnosis as CREST syndrome. Every letter in CREST stands for something. It made sense. C is for calcinosis (calcium deposits), R is for Raynaud's (constricted blood vessels in extremity vessels causing discoloration and numbness), E is for esophagitis (limp esophagus muscle), S is for sclerosis of the skin (hardening of the connective tissue primarily on the fingers and face). I didn't have the T yet but that came soon enough. The T is telangiectasia which means tiny blood vessels split open and cause red spots on the hands and face. This is one of the worst symptoms of all because it affects my appearance (Este Lauder concealer makeup works miracles).

The rheumatologist explained that CREST syndrome is a subset of scleroderma. The symptoms are a nuisance to deal with but not life threatening. I was happy to hear this. I was told by the rheumatologist that sometimes organ involvement happens. He went on to say I might be safe from experiencing organ involvement since I'd had CREST syndrome progressing over the past seventeen years and hadn't developed organ involvement. Usually organ involvement would develop within five or so years from the time your CREST syndrome symptoms first appear. So, I went on my merry way thinking I have a less serious version of scleroderma which was a good thing.

The rheumatologist wanted to see me every two months, but I didn't adhere to that. I didn't want to be so focused on this aspect of my life. It took too much time and energy. I was too busy. Dealing with CREST syndrome, I could handle on my own. As the doctor said, they are nuisance symptoms rather than life threatening. I wanted to continue living life.

I noticed another symptom cropped up which relates to the letter S in CREST, which stands for sclerosis. My face was tightening and my mouth was shrinking. Having work done by a dentist is probably the most uncomfortable of anything relating to CREST syndrome for me. There is no elasticity in the face and mouth and there is constant tingling. Every minute of every day you are aware of this feeling. I'd look at myself in the mirror and think, is my face changing? It was changing, but I was trying to tell myself that it wasn't too bad. I didn't really understand what was causing CREST syndrome at this point, and I didn't want to know. All I knew from the rheumatologist was it is a subset of scleroderma. I understood that to mean not as serious as full scleroderma.

I was working this particular day, 9-11-2001, when we saw planes go into the twin towers in Manhattan on TV at our DC office and other planes were headed for DC, possibly the White House. We were only one block away from the White House. Not too long afterwards, we were asked to evacuate the building by the U.S. Secret Service. Our company was located within the Secret Service perimeter of the White House. It was big. It took forever to get home. It was chaos in downtown DC. I remember saying to myself, "Is this what war sounds like?" There were sirens and emergency vehicles everywhere. We were all stunned walking in the streets not really knowing what was next. I remember my brother Tom was working in Manhattan which was another chaotic scene on an even bigger scale. We both made it through OK, but it was an experience that will never be forgotten. Eventually, our office moved to Arlington, Virginia to get away from the disruption. There were many scares subsequent to 9-11. This event took my mind off CREST syndrome that's for sure.

A new phenomenon cropped up with my physical condition. I would cough continuously while I had conversations with people. I remember a fellow I worked with would always feel bad that I couldn't talk without coughing. The more I talked the more I coughed. I actually remember coughing quite a bit while I was still in Southern New Hampshire before I moved to Maryland. People in New Hampshire whom I worked with thought it was an exercise induced cough. It made sense to me. I was a very active person.

I started to feel a little short-breathed though which I didn't like, especially at night when settling down to sleep. My PCP prescribed Advair which is an inhaler. I would often get bronchitis in the winter. He treated me with antibiotics. After so many treatments of antibiotics, my PCP requested that I go to a pulmonologist for consultation. This was in 2003. The pulmonologist did several breathing tests and evaluations. He didn't say I had scleroderma but he did suggest I go to the scleroderma center at Johns Hopkins in Baltimore just for a consultation. He gave me the scleroderma specialist's name and phone number. I never went.

The pulmonologist suggested I switch the inhaler to Spiriva instead of Advair. Spiriva doesn't have steroids. Advair does have steroids. He didn't prescribe any new treatment for me, and I didn't sense there was anything real critical happening so I figured I was OK to carry on with CREST syndrome, on my own. I was a little confused why I was coughing when CREST syndrome didn't cover such a symptom. I just didn't want to get caught up in dealing with a medical condition that so far didn't hold me down. Denial.

I was having a good time with my life, workwise and personally; the walks in DC, the fun dinners, the theatre, sites. There is so much to see and do in the DC, Maryland, and Virginia areas. I should mention Delaware, too, with the Eastern Shore. Two friends and I had such a fun time on a long weekend at the Eastern Shore one year. We laughed so hard we were crying.

I met many interesting people throughout the years. I even won awards I am proud of. Through work I was giving presentations periodically to large groups of people at this point, which didn't come easily to me, but it was part of the job. I learned how important it is to prepare, prepare, and prepare some more. Doing my homework was the key. I remember on a trip to Colorado I was scheduled to deliver a presentation to about 400 of our business partners, and I thought, "I forgot my concealer makeup that I used for Telangiectasia (the T in CREST that finally surfaced)." I was panicked. I had the hotel personnel suggesting places I could go to purchase concealer. There weren't many. It was such an ordeal. I ended up finding it in my luggage, and the presentation went smoothly. Thank God. I stressed over giving presentations, but the more I did them the better it got. Preparation really is the key for so many things in life.

I took on being the president of the townhouse association where I lived in Maryland. It was a small association of seventy-six townhomes to which we paid a common fee. The overall community consisted of townhomes and single-family homes so there was a homeowners association that we all paid into for common fee as well. I enjoyed working with the seven board members of our townhouse association as well as the members of the homeowners association board. It was a new learning experience. Both associations had their own set of covenants and by-laws that were exactly the same. It was kind of an odd setup, but the reason for giving the townhouse association separate documents is that the townhomes owned their two streets (not thru-streets) whereas the single-family home streets were owned by the county. It appeared to me as I took this role on that the associations were somewhat disconnected. One of the things I realized was that the homeowners association had delegated the compliance of their covenants to the townhouse association board to manage for the townhomes. The previous townhouse board had allowed this to happen. I took it upon myself to change that with the help of the townhouse board.

We involved our legal counsel to make sure our bases were covered. It was discovered the homeowner association was required to handle all members equally (townhouses and single-family homes). I negotiated with the homeowners association to incorporate the townhomes in their normal process for compliance, communications, everything. It was challenging. They had operated a certain way for many years, and I was changing that. I really enjoyed this challenge. We worked out a process that both associations could live with. It brought the two associations closer together and promoted consistency between the two. After all, we were all one community. Yah, there were a few complainers that the boards had to deal with occasionally, but I personally offered to deal with these people in the townhouse association. I liked the challenge of turning these people around or work with them to fix a problem. I made them part of the solution rather than part of the problem. I loved turning their perspective around. Maybe I wouldn't have liked it if there were frequent issues. Thankfully, the issues were minimal. Overall this was a great life experience.

5

RUNNING ON EMPTY

In September 2007, after eight years with my current company, a job offer came to me at a small consulting company in DC. I had dropped a seed to the vice president of the company at a conference figuring what do I have to lose? I thought, "I've worked for large companies so far, it would be interesting to work for a small company; a new experience." I received an offer a few months later and I happily accepted. I was back in DC but in the Georgetown area.

In November, two months after I started though, I had an episode while walking the few blocks uphill to the Dupont Circle metro stop, on my way home, my usual commute routine. I was walking with a colleague up the hill, and when I got to the top, I thought I was going to collapse. I told the colleague to continue on. I need to rest for a minute. Luckily there were café tables and chairs around and a small band playing. I just rested.

Normally, I walked by myself up that hill to the train so I could go at my own pace. There were stone walls along the way where I could rest as needed. If a colleague was leaving work at the same time as me, I would start out walking and then say, "Oh, I need to stop at CVS for something." This allowed me to be able to make it up that hill by myself. It worked most of the time. But this one time I forgot the CVS strategy. I fought to keep up with this colleague the whole way up the hill. After I rested several minutes, I was OK to continue on.

It just so happened, it was the last workday before Thanksgiving. I was heading to Connecticut to be with family for the holiday. While I was in Connecticut, my upper back was hurting so much. I took a lot of Motrin. I didn't know what was happening but it had my attention. I did think that walk uphill to the Dupont Circle metro stop might have had something to do with how I was feeling. I managed to get through the holiday weekend.

Soon after I arrived back in Maryland, I was in so much pain in my upper back I drove myself to the emergency room at eleven o'clock at night. They took an x-ray first and then a CT scan. I was told I have pleurisy and that I need to see a pulmonologist. They gave me pain medicine and sent me home at four o'clock in the morning. I drove myself home. I made an appointment with a pulmonologist soon after. He did tests and confirmed I have interstitial lung disease (ILD, pulmonary fibrosis) caused by scleroderma, and he could see the symptoms of scleroderma in my face and hands. He put me on sixty milligrams of prednisone and prescribed pain medicine as well.

He was very concerned. I remember him saying to me, "I feel like I've just turned on a movie, and I don't know if it's the beginning, the middle, or the end of the movie." I kept my composure. I really didn't feel very good. I guess I realized at this point organ involvement may have finally hit. Although I took a week off to get myself together, I went back to work. I had just started a new job, so I didn't have much time built up for vacation or being sick. During my commute I would feel the prednisone at work. It was as if I was breathing artificially by the way my breathing sounded. It was crackly. I started losing weight. But the prednisone seemed to be helping.

I remember one morning on my way to work I was at the Dupont Circle metro stop. The escalator at this stop is notorious for its length and steepness. I was on my way up the escalator. All of a sudden it stopped. I just looked up and thought, "How am I going to get to the top?" I was in the middle of the escalator. Walking down wouldn't do me any good. I had to go to work. It was dreadful.

I had to pull all my strength together to walk up the broken escalator. People were encouraging me and whispering in my ear you can do it. Take your time. I literally would take a step up and rest. I was holding back the tears. But I think I finally broke down. I just didn't have the lung capacity to walk up a steep escalator that was broken. I did finally make it to the top but I didn't want to have to do that again anytime soon. I rested when I got to the top until I felt strong enough to walk the few blocks to get to work.

Eventually I started taking a cab on the way up to the Dupont Circle metro stop at the end of the day. I didn't have the lung capacity to walk up the distance of that hill. I was able to walk down the few blocks to get to the office at the beginning of the day; the walk was on a decline, much easier for me. No problem. I did not want to give in to this disease.

I had my share of falls during my walks to work. Mostly I was in a rush but my coordination seemed slightly off. I ruined a suit from one of my falls. I got to work with blood all over my right knee. Another fall, I landed in the middle of an intersection. All traffic was stopped. It was so embarrassing. I had to really work on slowing down. Going downhill it was so easy to walk fast. On the way back up the hill at the end of the day it was a whole different story.

Another fall was a little more involved. I was on my way into Chipotle's for a burrito bowl, and I misjudged the curb. I fell flat on my face on concrete. Blood was everywhere. I remember the impact of the fall was my nose and mouth. My hands had my pocketbook and a bottle of water in them. It happened so fast I couldn't break the fall. The lady behind me was startled. She rushed in to Chipotle's to get paper towels. I went over and sat on the ground under a tree. It was a beautiful day luckily. I tried to stop shaking and get a grip on what just happened. I knew I had to go to the doctor because the blood kept coming. I ended up driving myself to a walk-in clinic with a cloth over the lower part of my face. They took an x-ray of my nose. I don't know how it didn't break, but it didn't. I needed four stitches on my lip. I was bruised everywhere. It happened on a Saturday. I went to work on Monday looking pretty bad but I felt OK. My appearance shocked the people at work, but within a few days my face was looking better. I had a wedding to go to soon after so I needed to be healed by then. I was healed enough to be inconspicuous.

In retrospect, when I was working for my previous company on Fourteenth and G Street, this one day we had a fire drill. We were on the fifth floor. When we were told we could go back in the building, our division lawyer said to me let's go up the stairs it will be quicker than waiting to get the elevator with all the people in line waiting. I said, "OK, that's a good idea."

A few others had the same idea. Well, I started struggling at the fourth floor. I was weak. The lawyer said "Where's your stamina?"

I said, "I don't know." I barely made it to the fifth floor. Signs were happening for a while.

6

SCLERODERMA

In February 2008, I met a fellow, through my Godmother, who has scleroderma. Andrew grew up in the same town where I grew up, in Massachusetts. We met for dinner one night during one of his business trips in the Maryland-DC area. His experience in 2000 was with the diffuse type of scleroderma affecting primarily his skin, joints, and his kidneys. He went into acute renal failure caused by scleroderma and almost died. His blood pressure was off the charts and he went into a coma. It was traumatic. He was in the hospital for thirteen days. The doctors put him on dialysis and miraculously after six months he was able to stop the dialysis. His other scleroderma symptoms even became inactive over time.

Meeting him was very helpful. He's a very inspiring individual. As a motivational speaker, you can imagine he had a positive influence on me. He told me I need to see a scleroderma specialist. A scleroderma specialist is a rheumatologist that specializes in scleroderma. So I looked around online and found a well-renowned hospital in Maryland, Johns Hopkins, has a Scleroderma Center. Johns Hopkins is only about forty minutes away from my house. I thought, "How fortunate that is." Maybe this was the reason for the move to Maryland. I recalled the conversation with the pulmonologist I saw initially in 2003 who recommended I go to Johns Hopkins Scleroderma Center for a consultation. This was during my denial stage. Oh well. I pulled out the note I saved with the contact information. I got an appointment in May with a scleroderma specialist, Dr. Laura Hummers.

I learned there are two types of scleroderma, localized and systemic. Localized scleroderma is more common in children. I won't elaborate on the localized version of scleroderma as I have the systemic version, but I wanted to acknowledge it in case someone wants to research it more.

The two types of systemic scleroderma are *limited* scleroderma and *diffuse* scleroderma. CREST as mentioned in an earlier chapter is an older designation for limited scleroderma but it has fallen out of favor as a terminology. The medical field refers to limited scleroderma to define this syndrome. You either have limited scleroderma or diffuse scleroderma. Limited scleroderma is no less serious than diffuse scleroderma despite the name. The main difference between the two types is the diffuse scleroderma often presents itself with aggressive disease at the onset and can burn out after two years. More often the damage is done in the first two years of disease. Limited scleroderma more often starts off insidiously and lung involvement develops in ten to twenty years after disease onset. It is the patients with overlap of both limited and diffuse scleroderma who often have combined features of both diseases (I happen to be one of them).

In general, scleroderma is a rare, chronic auto-immune disease. Approximately 300,000 Americans are diagnosed with the disease and there are still many looking for answers and coping with a variety of symptoms. Scleroderma literally means "hard skin." However, the

disease is better defined as being character-
ized by a hardening or thickening of the body's
connective tissue. Scleroderma causes your
immune system to go on auto-pilot and produce an overabundance of connective tissue in
your body for no reason, thus the hardening
or thickening.

Connective tissue is present all throughout our bodies to keep the configuration of our
internal bodily systems intact. With this disease, the immune system is on auto-pilot. It
produces extra connective tissue anywhere in
your body, again, for no reason. There's no
known methodology for where the connective
tissue is produced. When you have too much
connective tissue in your body, it causes hav-
oc with your bodily systems and makes them
function less efficiently.

There is no known cure for scleroderma,
and the cause of scleroderma is unknown.
Significant progress is being made in treatments for many scleroderma patients. The
positive message is that more and more research is being done to find improved treatments, and hopefully, the cause and cure will
be discovered eventually through grants and
donations.

Note, *systemic sclerosis* (Ssc) is another
name for scleroderma and *collagen* is another

name for connective tissue. One would think extra collagen is a good thing. People get injections of it to make them look younger. Not so, when there is too much of it. Your body can't handle it. Your tissue is too thick.

The specialist confirmed I do in fact have systemic Sclerosis with interstitial lung disease caused by scleroderma. She arranged for me to have a procedure called a bronchoscopy to see how bad my lungs were. From the expression on her face I knew it wasn't good. I was a little in shock. I remember asking her is this something I need to tell my family. I did not have any family in Maryland. She said it would be a good idea. She was very encouraging and compassionate. I knew I was in the right care.

She did not want me on Prednisone so I had to get off it gradually. My understanding is that prednisone has not been shown to have much clinical efficacy in slowing down or reversing the damage done by this disease, and it can precipitate a scleroderma renal crisis in diffuse patients. She put me on Cytoxan which is a form of chemotherapy, but I couldn't tolerate it. It made me nauseous and weak and I had to drink two liters of water per day to avoid bladder cancer.

After three months of Cytoxan she tried another option. She put me on CellCept. Cell-Cept is a medication primarily used to suppress the immune system from rejecting a transplanted organ. The idea for scleroderma patients is that CellCept will suppress the immune system from producing the overabundance of connective tissue in the body for no reason. I was on the maximum dose a person can be on, 3000 milligrams per day.

I lost several pounds in the process. I went from a size six to a size four to a size two, and then I used safety pins for my pants and skirts so that I didn't have to start buying size zero. I had a few size zeroes but managed to work with the size twos. It was expensive because I was working all this time in a professional environment and needed to dress professionally.

In retrospect, I don't know how I coped so well, but I was doing it. My clients didn't notice. I hid my situation well. I eventually made management aware of what I was experiencing. I waited as long as I could to tell them. They were so cooperative and understanding. I was very thankful for that. My thought was there is no known cause, no cure, and the treatment for my situation is scant. I was determined to fight this condition.

I kept thinking it is fun working for a small company. The environment was more personable and less political than that of a large company. This was nice for a change. I know management was happy with my work. They even let me work from home three days a week. This was such a big help. Being on CellCept, I went for blood tests often and pulmonary rehab after work a few times a week to help with my physical stamina. I saw Dr. Hummers at the Scleroderma Center every three months.

7

POWER OF ENERGY HEALING

Breathing took up so much of my energy. Interestingly, in 2009, I was introduced to an energy healer, Mary, by my tax accountant, Baljit. Baljit is originally from India. I really believe meeting her was meant to be. She introduced me to a highly skilled and powerful energy healer. Energy healing is something I had never been exposed to. But I was open to it. Here I have a condition that has no known cause, no cure, and little treatment. "I have nothing to lose and everything to gain," I thought.

Mary is a master healer, teacher and instructor for Reiki, Integrated Energy Therapy, and other energy healing modalities. There is a great deal of training that you go through to become a healer/teacher/instructor. Energy healing is considered both holistic and spiritual. They dovetail one another. Holistic healing means treatment of the whole person taking into account mental and social factors, rather than just the physical symptoms of a disease.

The spiritual component gets in touch with our soul or consciousness through meditation. Often times, people refer to mind and body but forget about the spirit. From my experience with energy healing, spirit is equally as important as mind and body. Tapping into the body's own frequencies (energy) as a type of alternative medicine is being taken seriously by health practitioners trained in both eastern and western modalities of medicine. I have learned the medical field is becoming much more respectful toward energy healing as a complimentary treatment. Dr. Oz's wife is a Reiki master. I think that is interesting. I do believe certain people are gifted to heal others whether it's energy healing, medical treatments, or a combination.

Of course, I believe God is ultimately in control, but God gave us free will to utilize energy healers and the medical field to help us. We have the ability to make things better too by surrounding ourselves with positive energy and exuding it at the same time. We may not always understand, but by having faith in God, it gives me strength to deal with whatever comes my way. I believe all my life experiences are for the growth of my soul. I learned the human body includes seven major Chakras which are energy centers that continually spin in our body. These spinning vortices or energy centers receive, assimilate and express our vital life energy. They are connected to certain areas and organs of the body. It is believed by many these energy centers are linked to the universe, God, our creator.

The Chakras can become blocked. They are supposed to spin in harmony with each other. Meditation is powerful for balancing chakras. It does take practice. Mary's work with me has helped balance my chakras and helped keep me as strong as possible in dealing with scleroderma. From my experience, connecting with my soul has given me such comfort. You leave your ego at the door and allow your soul to come through.

Mary sometimes channels the healing angels through Integrated Energy Therapy. She's done this with me. Through this process, I learned I have a guardian angel named Rebecca. I was especially surprised to hear my guardian angel is named Rebecca as I was given a book when I was very young called Rebecca of Sunnybrook Farm that has mysteriously been with me my whole life. I forgot what the book was about but it stayed with me over the years for some reason. It is a hard cover book and the binding is all falling apart. When I read it as an adult after I found out my guardian angel is Rebecca, I loved it. It's a classic story about positive living. I really believe there are no coincidences. I looked this book up on the internet and learned it is a significant book for both children and adults. I have the 1960 version of the book. It cost one dollar back then. You should check it out.

There are many things I could talk about here from my experiences with Mary but the most notable is that the angel guides said early on I was going to go through a medical procedure (they didn't say what type). They said it will happen swiftly, do not back down. I believe energy healing has given me strength and inner peace especially to deal with scleroderma but even in my daily life. My faith in God has become so powerful through this energy healing process. I feel very connected and have continual hope. The field of energy is fascinating to me. I hope to keep learning about it.

8

SAYING GOODBYE TO THE CITY

Out of the blue I was approached by a colleague, Dianne, I worked with in the past who wanted to hire me at a large company. I was so excited. I explained what I was dealing with pertaining to my health but that I was managing the condition and functioning quite well. I told her I had to go for blood tests and rehab periodically. She knew I was a fighter and said, "We can make it work."

I interviewed with her boss, and I remember he came to the lobby to get me. We had to go up a flight of stairs to his office and funny thing is he gave me the option of us taking the elevator. I said, "Oh, no. Stairs are fine."

I knew though I might get winded, which I did, but I hid it to the point he didn't notice. They made me an offer. This was in September 2009. I accepted. I accepted this offer because it was closer to home, and it actually was the next step I had wanted to make in my career. It was a short commute and they had their own parking lot right at their building. I always enjoyed working with this colleague. She was a mentor and my best advocate for many years. She brought out the best in me. She challenged me. We had some great memories from the past, both personally and business related. I worked for the small consulting company for two years. I couldn't have asked for a better experience, but now on to another new adventure. No more public transportation and city. I had a feeling this move might be my last move, where I retire. Don't laugh or... go ahead and laugh if you want. As I write about this journey, I realize how determined I was to try and conquer this disease, to *will* it away.

I have to tell you a little story that I hate to admit about my last days at this consulting company. I was putting a lot of effort into preparing and transitioning my client files and actions so someone could come in and take over. This one night I worked late until about 9:30 p.m., and I thought, "Now I have to take a cab up the hill to the Dupont Circle metro stop because I can't walk up the hill anymore. Then I have to take the train to the parking garage, get my car, and drive home. I didn't have it in me. I decided to take a cab all the way home from DC instead. It wasn't inexpensive, but I was just too tired to take on the commute. I grabbed something light to eat when I got home and then settled in for the night. The next day I worked from home which was good since I worked so late at the office the night before. When I looked out my window in the kitchen my car wasn't in my parking space. It was stolen. I called the insurance company and the police and reported it. The insurance company advised me to get a car rental while we resolved the case. I was all stirred up about the whole thing. I told some family members and my neighbor and friends about it. It was awful.

Anyway, the next day I had to go to DC again so I drove in my rental car to the parking garage. I even called one of my friends at work on my way to the garage and told her about my car being stolen. When I got to the parking garage I parked right where I usually park. To my dismay, as I was parking the rental car I saw my car. It wasn't stolen! I was shocked. I forgot I had taken a cab the whole way home two nights prior and left my car in the parking garage. That is pretty bad.

I continued on to get on the train for DC. I had things to do. Great, now I have to call the insurance company and tell them my car wasn't stolen, it was a mishap. The insurance company thought I was crazy. Trying to explain my way out of this one was not easy. I called the police and informed them as well, not to mention everyone else I told. The police wouldn't void the police report unless I met the police where my car is to show it's no longer stolen. I had to wait until they could meet me. This wasn't their biggest priority.

We made arrangements to meet that night and took care of business. I asked my neighbor if she could help me get two cars out of the parking garage at her convenience. I drove home in one car and then my neighbor and I drove back in her car so I could pick up the other car. The joke's on me! I said to myself, it just goes to show how hard I was working to keep up with everything. We all had some good laughs about it none the less. You have to keep your sense of humor.

My scleroderma specialist, Dr. Hummers, was happy to hear I didn't have to commute into DC anymore. I was pretty happy too. I felt really safe with her. I knew I was in good hands. I finally got off the sixty milligrams of Prednisone. It took some time but the transition went well.

I continued on the CellCept she had put me on. I think I mentioned earlier the purpose of having me on the CellCept was to attempt to slow down my immune system from over-producing connective tissue in my body for no reason and especially now in my lungs. I was still able to have a social life to an extent. Work tired me out somewhat, but I always put in a full day's work and some. I was managing to handle everything with my home. I did have someone come to clean my house (the heavy chores) when it became a challenge for me. It was a three-level Townhouse. I also had groceries delivered by the Peapod service.

I loved my home in Maryland. It was tucked back on a cul-de-sac surrounded by park land. It was very private and quiet even though it was so close to the city.

I actually put in long days at this new job, but it was satisfying work. We were so busy. It was a federal contractor environment selling to the U.S. Army; very demanding but challenging and interesting. Work to me was never just a job. It was an opportunity to learn, grow, and reap the rewards. I met a lot of nice people there.

It was hard to find time to go to the rehab center and get blood tests, but I managed it because I realized I have no choice. No more denial. There was someone at the rehab center with scleroderma, Nancy, and it was comforting to talk with her. Thankfully for her, she didn't have organ involvement but she had plenty of other symptoms. The director at the rehab center, Susan, was a Godsend. She, along with so many of the staff there, encouraged me so much.

By Spring of 2010, only eight months after I started the new job, my physical body was seriously declining. I remember being in the hallway with colleagues talking about business matters. I would start to feel light-headed and need to sit down. I didn't want to make it obvious, so I would say I just remembered I have to make a phone call. It got to the point where my manager noticed me struggling to keep up. She suggested I go out on short-term disability (STD). I guess I couldn't hide it anymore.

My initial response was, "No I think I'm good." But the more I paid attention, the more I realized she's right. I'm worn out. Talking even depleted my energy.

9

OXYGEN IN A TANK

My niece, Meghan, came to see me for Easter. She was living in Virginia at the time and her fiancée was away on a hockey trip. He played in the AHL. We had a nice visit. I remember giving her an Easter basket. It was fun making an adult basket. She was twenty-three at the time. We went together to Bed Bath and Beyond to purchase a shower bench because I was having trouble standing in the shower. It was a big help.

I went out on short-term disability in June 2010. I was putting a lot into preparing a seamless transition for someone to take over and be able to continue without me being there. This was eight months after I started the job. Once I left I was shocked to discover how bad off I was. It hit me I had been running on pure adrenaline for so long. I knew at this point there was no going back to work. I had to let go. There was no question in my mind. It's like the flu, you know when you have the flu you have to call out sick.

I remember in November 2010 asking Dr. Hummers if a lung transplant would be a possibility in the future. She said transplant would be the next step. I learned later she had me on CellCept because you have to exhaust every possible treatment avenue. Transplant is the last resort.

I took the train to Connecticut for the Christmas holiday. I was pretty thin. You could see it in my face, but I managed. I wasn't strong enough to travel for Thanksgiving too so my friend Ginnie invited me to her Thanksgiving gathering. I really appreciated and enjoyed it.

Some people would say why are you staying in Maryland? Don't you want to be closer to your family? I thought about that, but I was so close to Johns Hopkins Scleroderma Center in Maryland that I didn't think it was the right thing to move. I had researched Connecticut where most of my family lived, and there was only one scleroderma specialist at the University of Connecticut that I could find and no lung transplant center in case I needed a transplant. My gut told me I was in the right place. Not to mention Maryland was home. I wasn't emotionally or physically ready to pack up and move at that point.

In January 2011, not too long after I got back to Maryland from Connecticut, I was back in the hospital. This time I went by ambulance. I decided not to drive myself. I was in so much pain in my upper back again (worse than the time in 2007). I was taken right in. I remember the nurse listened to my lungs and her reaction was "Oh God." They did a CT scan and found the results showed the connective tissue in the lungs was much worse when they compared it to my CT scan in 2007. They admitted me into the hospital, and I was there for five days. I was sent home with oxygen; nineteen hours on oxygen and five hours off. My neighbor, Jackie, picked me up. I am very grateful for all her support through the years in Maryland. She was a good neighbor and friend. We trusted each other with our house keys too. I was instructed to follow up with my scleroderma specialist.

Meanwhile, a couple of weeks prior to me going in the hospital, I received a call from my best friend in high school, JoAnn, whom I hadn't seen in years. My mother had bumped into her at the grocery store up in Connecticut. They got talking. My mom told her about my health situation. She wanted to come see me. She called me. We talked, and she booked a train ride pretty quickly. I was so excited. We had connected one other time when I was divorced up in New Hampshire. It was like no time had passed. We had such a good time. But somehow we lost touch again.

My sister, Pat, called JoAnn to let her know I was in the hospital and getting home right before she planned on arriving. Pat wanted to give JoAnn the option of going to Maryland or not. It was the right thing to do. JoAnn still wanted to come, but she wanted to make sure it wouldn't be too much for me. Pat suggested that she call me. So JoAnn and I talked. She asked me if I want her to still come. I said I think I do want you to come. I was in good spirits and couldn't wait for her visit. JoAnn and I had so many laughs my stomach hurt. In fact, she postponed her trip for a few more days. I did everything I could to be strong and positive. Since I could be off oxygen for five hours a day, I used these five hours for when I went out. I was so happy to see her. She went to the follow up visit with me to see Dr. Hummers. I remember she cut up apples and sprinkled the apple sections with lemon first and then cinnamon sugar. They tasted so good. JoAnn's visit was so good for me. She lifted me up.

Dr. Hummers and I talked about the oxygen situation. I didn't take it with me to the appointment since I had those five hours I didn't need to be on it. She said I would argue you need to be on the oxygen whenever you are exerting yourself, for example, coming to a doctor's appointment. She said, "Frankly, you need to be on oxygen all the time."

By March 2011, I was due to see Dr. Hummers again. So I went to the appointment. My sister Nancy who lived in Florida willingly came up to Maryland and went to the appointment with me. I was so happy to have her with me. I had a PET scan done of my chest the week before because there was a dense mass at the bottom of my right lung. I was going to get the results at this appointment. The purpose of this test was to rule out cancer. I was a wreck. Thankfully there was no cancer. It was the connective tissue.

I asked Dr. Hummers, "How sick do you have to be before you can qualify for a transplant?"

She responded, "You are there." It brought tears to my eyes. I had declined so rapidly. I had wrestled with scleroderma for many years, but this stage of the disease was very trying. I was almost ready to give up, but I dug down deep for strength. Johns Hopkins Comprehensive Transplant Center wouldn't do the lung transplant because I had scleroderma, too much risk with the esophageal issues. This was concerning. Nancy and I went home thinking about what was ahead. My sisters Nancy and Pat talked. Pat got on the phone with me and said you are coming to Connecticut to stay with John and me for a while. Get ready we're driving down to pick you up.

I had to get my clothes together and make arrangements to have oxygen in Connecticut. Having oxygen means having a concentrator in the home, a medium size machine that is an electric device. It produces oxygen by concentrating the oxygen that is already in the air and removing other gases. This method is less expensive, easier to maintain, and doesn't require refilling. There are also portable tanks or cylinders of steel that hold smaller amounts of oxygen for when going out of the home. You can fill a cylinder by using the concentrator or the vendor that provides the concentrator can provide prefilled cylinders. At rehab you would bring your portable oxygen tank with you and then hook your nasal cannula up to a wall connection for oxygen so you don't waste the oxygen in your portable tank. You would do the same for doctor appointments as well. It's extremely important to not allow any form of fire in the house while oxygen is in the house. No candles, and so on. Being on oxygen was a humbling experience.

I think back now, my sense of taste was gone. Corn flakes tasted like paper. I noticed I couldn't see out of my eye glasses any more either. I thought, "I must need a stronger prescription." Maybe it would be a good idea to get my eyes checked before I have a transplant. Get it out of the way. In August my mom took me to the eye appointment. After my exam the doctor said my sight completely changed so he updated my prescription. I didn't wear my eye glasses again until well after my transplant but I figured at least I will have them for when I want to use them. As it turned out, when I did try to use my reading glasses several weeks after the transplant, I couldn't see out of them. I went back to the eye doctor at that point and had another eye exam. He compared my exam results to my last couple of exam results. He said my prescription is more like my prescription before my last exam. In other words, being on oxygen affected my eye sight. The eye doctor was very intrigued by this and said he wanted to share this finding with other eye doctors in the field. The lack of oxygen can impact eye sight. We both thought that it's better to wait until after a transplant to have an eye exam if possible. So the lack of oxygen affected my taste buds, my eye sight, and my sense of balance too (why I was falling or getting light-headed while standing).

Throughout this difficult time, I never lost my faith in God, ever. I always had hope.

10

FRIENDS AND FAMILY

It was the end of March. I had to decide where to have the transplant. My family and I thought Boston University Medical Center was a good option for a transplant. Most of my family members are in Connecticut and New Hampshire. Turns out Boston University Medical Center wouldn't take on the risk of doing a lung transplant on a scleroderma patient for similar reasons as Johns Hopkins; too much risk with the esophageal issues. It was troubling that certain lung transplant centers were not willing to perform a lung transplant on a scleroderma patient. The lung transplant center in Boston recommended University of Pittsburgh in PA or Inova Fairfax Hospital in Virginia. I looked into Inova Fairfax in Virginia. My family and I agreed it could work if I had it done in Virginia. Dr. Hummers thought it was the best option too. It was a close enough drive back and forth from my home in Maryland to Virginia. She immediately put my name in to Inova Fairfax Hospital for a lung transplant.

Meanwhile I am now at my sister Pat's house in Connecticut with oxygen and all. I stayed for two months through the end of May. It was a memorable time. My sister and her family made my stay so comfortable. It was not easy on them. I was basically useless. I could take a shower if I had a seat in the shower. They got one for me. I was done for the day after the shower. I was very underweight, ninety-six pounds. Dr. Hummers said, "You will need to gain some weight as part of the criteria for having a transplant. You have to be strong enough to get through the surgery."

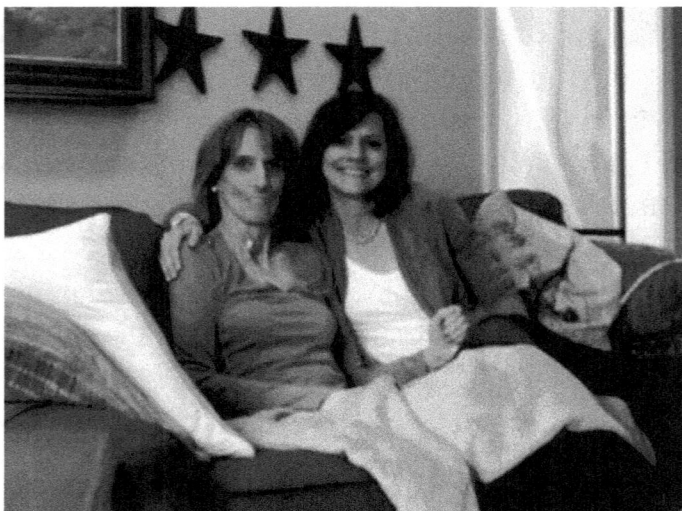

Figure 1. Before transplant surgery with my sister Pat

Pat and I set out to help me gain weight. She made milkshakes and lots of good food. She is a great cook. I remember being in the family room on the couch with my oxygen. I was admiring the plant on a cabinet between the kitchen and the family room. There is a mirror above the cabinet. I happened to look in the mirror. Pat who just made a milkshake was drinking the left over bit of milkshake right from the blender after she had poured the milkshake in a big glass for me. It was so funny. She really looked like she enjoyed it. I caught her doing that a couple of times. Another good memory was her capturing on video a family of robins making a nest, the mother laying the eggs and sitting on them until they hatched. She also captured the baby robins from the time they hatched until they left the nest one by one. There were three baby robins. It was unbelievable to watch this video. We learned a lot about robins. The video should have been put up on YouTube.

I remember another time the three of us were in their family room on a Friday night contemplating watching a movie. We decided on the movie.

John said, "I think I'll have a beer."

Pat said, "Maybe I'll have a glass of wine."

I said, with oxygen being fed in through my nose, "I'll take a pain pill."

We all laughed. The pain pills were an occasional relief because there were times when I overexerted myself, for example, walking down the stairway and after a delay of a minute or so I would be gasping for air. Anyway, I can't thank Pat and John and their kids enough for having cared for me those two months. They took me for blood tests when I needed them. I gained a few pounds too. We reminisce every year. Around this time, I heard from the transplant center at Inova Fairfax while in Connecticut. They wanted to see me for an evaluation appointment in June. I think it was the fifteenth. So at the end of May, my sister, Pat, and my brother-in-law John and my mom took me back to Maryland.

My sister, Nancy, and her husband, Joe, arrived in Maryland from Florida in time to meet us at my house. The plan was for Nancy and my mom to stay with me and go to the transplant center with me for the June appointment. Joe went back to Florida. He had to work. John and Pat went back to Connecticut as they had to work too. The three of us, Mom, Nancy, and me, would take one step at a time. We learned I needed to have a lot of medical tests done, and I had to continue my rehab. Rehab was really important to keep up whatever strength I had so I could be strong enough to get through the surgery. The tests were important to make sure I was healthy enough to get through the surgery. I needed to keep my weight up too because you lose weight from not being able to breathe and then you also lose it as a result of the surgery.

The three of us were busy. I don't know what I would have done without them. The transplant center gave us a whole list of tests that had to be done. We wanted to get them done in as short a time period as possible. The sooner the tests were completed the sooner I would know if I could be put on the lung transplant list. This ordeal was called the qualification process.

At the June appointment the transplant clinic drew twenty two tubes of blood. I was stunned. I just kept quiet and let them do their thing. I knew I had to go with the flow. Nancy, my mom and I got through many of the requested tests. I appreciated their help so much. They were very caring and giving. Feeding me and driving me all over for the various tests and rehab while being away from their homes was such a big sacrifice. I hoped having each other was helpful for them since I couldn't offer much. I was in such a weakened state. They were in Maryland for several weeks. All the tests results were good so far, thankfully.

In July my niece was getting married up in New Hampshire. There was a wedding shower my mom needed to be at. Nancy was generous enough to stay in Maryland with me while my mother went to the shower, which was another big sacrifice on Nancy's part. My brother Tom came down from Connecticut to pick my mother up. God bless him. Then the wedding came. I talked with my friend, JoAnn, who I had reconnected with from high school. She said she could come for a week while all were at the wedding. So she took the train down from Connecticut. It was so hard for me to depend on people. That might have been the hardest thing I had to deal with in retrospect. JoAnn and I managed to have such a fun time. She was very positive and encouraging. She had a way of picking my spirits up. She took me to an all day visit at Inova Fairfax for a series of tests. This day turned out to be hilarious. I have to tell you this story.

Off we go to Inova Fairfax Hospital in Virginia for the series of tests. It was complicated. According to the instruction sheet, some tests were color coded orange in one area of the hospital, and other tests were color coded green for another area of the hospital. The hospital was like a large airport. JoAnn made pizza the night before, and we packed it to eat along with some other snacks for our jaunt. It was the kind of pizza that was good at room temperature or hot.

We entered the hospital and had to go up the elevator one floor. This was a problem. JoAnn has a phobia of elevators, won't go in them at any cost. So we agreed, I'll go up in the elevator and she can walk up the one flight of stairs. We'd meet at the top. I got off the elevator and saw a café right there, so I sat at one of the tables and waited for her. I had all the paperwork for my tests and my oxygen of course. She had her pocketbook, my pocketbook, a spare portable oxygen tank, and our lunch satchel. When she didn't come, I was concerned something might have happened on the way up the stairway. I hoped she was OK. It was now a little past my appointment for my first procedure. I figured, "She'll be here soon, no need to panic."

Well what happened is she got to the top of the stairs and saw elevators but no Linda. She was wondering what happened to me. She thought I must have gotten stuck in the elevator (she was so glad she didn't go in that elevator). A woman walked by and asked, "Are you lost?"

She said, "No, but my friend is." (She threw me under the bus.) Unfortunately the stairway JoAnn went up led to a different set of elevators. The woman asked her, "What are you trying to find?"

JoAnn didn't have any of the paperwork so she didn't know what to tell the woman. All she remembered was orange and green color coding. The woman was looking at her like she was crazy. JoAnn said, "Let me call my friend."

The woman said, "That's a good idea." So JoAnn called me. My phone rang but it was in my pocketbook on her shoulder. Next thing you know a woman came from around the corner and seemed all happy to see me. I thought she was the person looking for me to do the test procedure. It was the woman who was trying to help JoAnn find me. She went back around the corner and then out came JoAnn looking like a bag lady with all the stuff she was holding in her arms. I laughed so hard my stomach hurt. We both were hysterical. We called that our Lucy and Ethel moment (from the *I Love Lucy* TV show in the 1950s): "Lucy and Ethel Go to the Hospital."

A nurse proceeded to wheel me to my procedure pretty fast and JoAnn walked beside us. The procedure involved having a mask with a pretty large tube in my mouth. I had to breathe in and out for twelve minutes. JoAnn stayed in the waiting room. I have to say, I was laughing so much I had all I could do to keep the tube in my mouth and finish the test. I couldn't stop laughing. The rest of the tests went as planned.

It was a long day but we got everything done that we set out to do. I remember the last test at the end of the day was in the pulmonary center. There was a waiting room and people in it. We didn't know how long we would have to wait. JoAnn decided to go for a little walk, and she would meet me back there. I had just finished the test and went back to the waiting room. No sooner did I get out there when JoAnn returned. She told me a doctor had seen her in the hallway and asked her if she was a patient. She replied "No but I *will* be if I don't get out of here soon." The doctor just laughed and continued on his way. We laughed about the whole day all the way home. We still laugh about it.

At this point, I couldn't stand at the sink for more than fifteen to twenty seconds. For some reason it was more difficult to stand still than it was to walk. I couldn't walk much of a distance though. I barely had enough stamina to walk from my bed to my bathroom. It was a major undertaking to stand up and brush my teeth. I had to sit down halfway through to rest. I was basically limited to my bed for the most part. If I went downstairs for something, I would have to go slowly back up the stairs and rest midway. I remember I wasn't think-ing about the fact that I was dying. All I could think about was how can I keep going like this? I was so weak. All my energy went to struggling to breathe. My sister Pat came down for a few days when JoAnn left, and then Pat's daughter and son (my beloved niece Emily and nephew Dan) came down for the remaining few days. Emily and Dan took me to another all day visit at the hospital for more tests. That day went smoothly. My mother came back to stay with me after my niece and nephew left. My brother Tom made several trips back and forth from Connecticut to Maryland. He was so dependable to meet whatever the needs were.

My friend Debbi who lived locally offered to go with my mother and me to an appointment at the hospital where I was to meet the transplant team. Debbi was such an advocate for me. She knew what I was going through and could speak specifically about my limitations and struggles.

My neighbor and friend, Jackie, went with me to an all-day information day at the hospital. This was a pre-transplant information day where different members of the hospital came in to talk about the various phases of the transplant and post-transplant process. We enjoyed the learning experience together.

There was another test I had to have which involved testing the mobility of my esophagus muscle and seeing how well my esophagus worked with my stomach. This was an important test because it could be a show stopper for the transplant. The reason most lung transplant centers don't want to do a lung transplant on a scleroderma patient is that the lungs and the esophagus are so close together there can be risk that fluid will get into the lungs and cause a serious complication during and after the transplant.

My mom was with me again at this point and took me to this test. I remember it was pouring rain that day. It took a lot of courage for her to drive in the bad weather. We had to go to a different Johns Hopkins facility. They put a flexible metal hose-like instrument through my nose down my throat. I had to lie down and swallow a liquid they gave me several times while they took pictures of how well the liquid went down my esophagus. My poor mother could hear the noises I was making during this test. The door was open, and the waiting room was pretty close by. It was not a fun test.

Then I was hooked up to a remote monitor that I had to wear for twenty-four hours (at home) so they could monitor what I ate and when I ate it. I had to keep track on a piece of paper and go back the next day so they could remove the monitor. I was so anxious about the results of this test knowing the results would carry a lot of weight on determining the risk factor for doing the lung transplant. Not to mention it was the last test on my plate during the qualification process.

My mom and I decided to go for ice cream. It was a beautiful day and there were shops along with an ice cream shop and a restaurant connected to the medical building where I had been for my test. We found outdoor tables in a courtyard that was part of the restaurant. My mother bought our ice cream while I sat at the table with my oxygen still trying to recover from that test. We were enjoying our time so much. It was such a beautiful afternoon we decided to have dinner in the courtyard. We had crab cakes that were delicious. There's nothing wrong with having dinner after dessert! It was such a memorable time together.

My sister Sue came down at this point to help me. She took time off from work. She and my mom took me to the GI doctor in Virginia to discuss the results of the esophagus tests. He said he had seen worse. He was willing to give the OK for surgery. Worst case, we can use a feeding tube after surgery for a while if complications arise. That meant the test results would most likely be acceptable to the transplant team. Tears came to my eyes. It was such a release of stress. Sue also took me to Inova Fairfax Hospital to meet the surgeon and the pulmonologist. All the test results had come back acceptable to them. It was such an emotional and happy moment. Sue emphasized to the surgeon, "My sister has no quality of life. Hopefully the transplant can happen soon."

At this point in my journey, all the work that had to be done to get on the list was done. Their decision on whether to have a double lung transplant or a single was also made. They will do a single lung transplant. You can live with one lung. These decisions are made on a case by case basis. You have to wait longer for a double lung transplant because it's not often that two good lungs come along at the same time.

The surgeon showed me where I would be cut for the operation and explained some things to me. He was so confident, it gave me courage. I just needed to gain a couple more pounds before they would put me on the transplant list. The pulmonologist gave me a medication to stimulate my appetite. It worked. The qualification process was completed. This process took two-and-a-half long months. It was such a relief to be done with it.

Now I had to be put on the list. That took another couple of weeks. The processes that are involved are incredible. There are a few organizations that need to be notified and onboard because once you are put on the list, the transplant has to happen fast. Everyone has to be coordinated. I had to keep up with the rehabilitation therapy. As weak as I was, it would help in post-surgery. I had to eat the best I could so they couldn't tell me at the last minute I didn't weigh enough. I had to stay alive until the transplant.

I have such a great family and friends that helped me through everything. I am deeply grateful. This was not easy giving up their time to help me. It didn't help that most of them were living in Connecticut or Florida and had to travel to Maryland. Some had to take time off from work. They were the best tag team anyone could have ever hoped for. I will remember what they all did for me forever.

11

BREATHE

I got on the transplant list August 29. I remember on September 2, I went to rehab. It was a Friday. My mom took me as she would frequently do while she was with me. She actually grew to enjoy it. It was a social thing for her seeing some of the older ladies that were there rehabbing. I went three days a week. My mom even helped the workers wheel people in and out of the hospital. There were a few people who were in rehab preparing for a lung transplant too. The rehab center felt like my home away from home. On our way home from rehab that day we stopped at the grocery store and then continued home. We were sitting in the living room knitting lap blankets (my friend JoAnn had taught me how to knit when I was in Connecticut for those two months) talking about what we were having for dinner. I said, "Mom we have to get this transplant thing out of our minds. It could take months, years to be called for a transplant." We agreed.

Now that I'm reliving all this by writing about it, what would we have done if it really did take months or years to get the phone call? What a complicated thought. It didn't even enter my mind what we would do. I was barely thinking properly at this point. I was dying but I didn't give up hope for this transplant. I was so ready and willing to do it. My mother went to bed at her usual time, 8:00 p.m. I stayed up as I usually did. It was around midnight I decided to check my email. I was looking at my email and all of a sudden my phone rang. I'm thinking who would be calling me at this hour. It was a little concerning at 1:07 a.m.

I picked up the phone and it was my doctor at Inova Fairfax. They had a lung for me! I said, "Is this a joke?"

I thought to myself, "It has only been five days since I got on the transplant list."

She said, "No. How fast can you be here?"

She said one thing I have to tell you is that we haven't been able to find the family yet to perform a background check. The woman I called before you who was on the transplant list said she didn't want to go through with this donor. I got a twinge in my stomach. I took a deep breath and said, "Do you think I should do it? This is kind of scary."

She said, "Well, this happens sometimes. It doesn't mean the lung isn't good."

I thought back to that night I was with the energy healer, Mary, and the angel guides said, "You are going to have a medical procedure. It will happen swiftly, do not back down."

I took another deep breath. I immediately said to the doctor, "I will leave shortly. Thank you."

I went in the guest room and informed my mother. We pulled our overnight bags together. I contacted the limousine service I had pre-arranged for this very moment. I had tested the limousine service once I got on the transplant list and it worked, so even though I was shaking to death, I felt in my gut it would work. And it did. They picked my mom and me up, and we proceeded on our way to the hospital. By now it was around 2:00 a.m.

On the way to the hospital, my mom told me my brother Tom is on his way from Connecticut. I said, "Oh I better call him just to let him know there is a chance I could be sent home due to a problem with the donated organ. They call this a false alarm."

The way the process works, the doctor notifies the patient of the available organ in parallel with other doctors getting in touch with the donor family, detaching the organ from the donor, inspecting the organ and getting it to the patient. I'm oversimplifying the process. There is only so much time an organ can be out of a body. The lung has the shortest window of time, I believe. There are many aspects of the donated lung that are checked by the medical team to insure a successful transplant.

We got to the hospital a little after 2:30 a.m. The doctor had told me to ring the bell at the transplant center entrance where I went for my clinic visits. Tell the person your name and say you are here for a lung transplant. So I did. The person on the intercom said, "Yes, Ms. Edwards, we are waiting for you. Come up to room 256." (I think my recollection is correct on the room number.)

They let my mom and me in the door. It was so quiet and still at the hospital being two-thirty in the morning. Everyone was settled in for the night. We got up to the hospital room oxygen in hand, and a nurse was waiting for me. She had antiseptic soap and said, "Get in the shower. Wash everywhere including your hair."

I said," OK." Thank God there was a seat in the shower. I was exhausted after standing for a few seconds. When I got out of the shower I asked the nurse, Is it possible at this point I could be sent home because of a false alarm?"

She replied. "The doctors have all examined the lung, completely. It is ready to be put inside you."

So I called my brother and told him, "The lung is good!" I was so happy. Meanwhile my brother was well on his way to Maryland regardless. I lay in the hospital bed with my mom beside me waiting for the doctors to say they were ready for me.

I had a blood draw and a chest x-ray. Nurses were coming in and out for different things. I had to sign a release paper exempting the hospital of all the risks that are involved. I had no problem signing the document. I had signed this paper a couple of times previously during the pre-transplant process, so I knew what it said. I didn't even care at this point. My faith was (and still is) so strong. I knew it was in God's hands. I was OK with that. I remember an operating nurse John came in and was looking over my records. His back was facing me as he was at the counter looking at my paperwork. He said, "Gee, you are really healthy if it wasn't for the scleroderma." My mom and I chuckled, she said, "You are right."

We finally got the word the doctors are ready for me. As they wheeled me in to the operating room, my mom was walking next to us until we finally had to say goodbye. I said, "It's going to be alright Mom. It's in God's hands. See you soon. Love you."

It was Saturday, September 3, 2011. I had a right lung transplant. My brother Tom arrived five minutes after I went into the operating room. This was perfect timing to be with Mom. She was being so strong, eighty years young at the time. In retrospect, this whole experience was probably worse for her than it was for me. Well, I guess it was hard for both of us for different reasons.

I just remember feeling at peace with what was about to happen. I wasn't afraid to die. I knew I didn't want to live in the condition I was in any longer. Whatever was supposed to happen would happen. I was good.

The operating room was pretty typical. I had had major surgery before, so it wasn't surprising. The room was cool. I remember the nurse put a warm blanket on me. Many machines were around and lots of metal. It was very calm. The operating nurses and doctors were very comforting and focused. I felt safe. I had hope. I remember they wanted me to put my arms above my head. The right arm wouldn't go up. I had frozen shoulder, a condition that restricts the motion of the shoulder joint, which I had had for a while. I tried my best. They were satisfied.

The next thing I remember is waking up to pure darkness, eyes closed, and an angelic voice softly saying, "Everything is OK, Ms. Edwards, just relax, breathe normally. You are safe. I am here with you. You can breathe normally. You are doing great."

Finally I came to. I was in ICU. I was on the ventilator for twelve hours after surgery. The nurse, Ann Marie, said she had never in all her thirty years as a lung transplant nurse seen someone get off the ventilator so soon. It usually takes twenty-four to forty-eight hours. I was so medicated but I was coherent. I asked for something to drink. The nurse said she couldn't give me anything to drink but she could give me crushed ice cubes. Some of my family members were in the room with me. Nancy and her husband, Joe, my mom, and my bother Tom. I was feeling so good (the drugs). I remember my brother Joe calling me from New Hampshire, and I was talking to him and his family. I said, "Ooh, my chair just moved." I was so drugged up it felt like my chair was swaying even though it wasn't. I wasn't even in a chair, it was a bed.

It was a fun sensation but when you are so medicated, anything is fun. Anyway, it was good to see my family in the ICU. They were so supportive and there for me. It was comforting to have them near. I have to say being in the ICU reminded me of being in a war zone even though I didn't know what a war zone was like. That was my impression.

Nurses would go flying by the door rushing to get somewhere. Loud buzzers would go off. It was very hectic. There was always some emergency going on. ICU nurses' work is extraordinarily rigorous. I was completely taken aback. It takes a special type of person to do that line of work. A person regretfully passed away in the ICU while I was there.

I remember thinking about whose lung I received. Was it a woman or a man? How did the person die? Did this person die in a car accident? Was this person shot? You don't find out. This information is anonymous. Nurses can't say anything about the donor.

A person's height determines the right lung size. Blood type is another factor, and the third primary factor is severity of condition. Five years earlier the process for getting matched with a donated organ was you get on the list and you wait for your name to reach the top of the list along with blood type and size. Then the rule changed. Severity of condition became a key factor. I figure I must have been in bad shape since I was only on the list for five days. I was lucky for that rule change.

Timing is everything as they say. Dr. Hummers at Johns Hopkins Scleroderma Center knew precisely what time to put my name in to the Transplant Clinic at Inova Fairfax Hospital. She was extraordinary. When I thanked her at an appointment several months later, she said, "I was doing my job." All I can say is thank God for her.

It's pretty interesting how intricately the process comes together from the time the donor is pronounced brain dead to the time the organ is put in to the transplant patient. It's miraculous. I was on my deathbed. I had been down to ninety-six pounds, on oxygen, with a medical condition called scleroderma with lung involvement that has no cure, no known cause, and little treatment. I sometimes ask myself why I made it through. I know people that did not make it through their transplant. Why did I make it and they didn't?

My brother Tom relayed to me what the surgeon said after the surgery. Tom told me he started crying with joy when the surgeon came up to him in the waiting room and told him the surgery couldn't have gone better. "It was a perfectly healthy lung your sister received. I wanted to see that perfectly pink color and when I removed the clamp it filled up like a balloon. That is exactly what I look for".

I have a picture of the new lung in my body. There are permanent large stitches around it that will never dissolve. Fascinating. Something else that was amazing is that my right lung was in worse condition than my left lung. The Donor's right lung was the good lung. The donor's left lung wasn't useable. I got the advantage of having a perfect lung put inside me to replace my worst lung. The stars were aligned that's all I can say.

Tom left Maryland early Monday morning to get back to work and to be with his family in Connecticut. My mom and Nancy stayed on. My brother-in-law Joe went back to work in Florida as well.

Monday evening the ICU nurses transferred me to my own regular hospital room. I had been in the ICU for three days. A nurse took me by wheel chair to my new room. I remember it was about 10:00 p.m. and it was on a different floor. I had my belongings on my lap and some of the nurse's items. It was a fun ride. We went pretty fast. I hadn't had that much fun in a while. We were laughing. I had a catheter in me that I was anxious to get rid of. But I have to admit, the thought of walking to the bathroom was a monumental task. My arms and legs were seriously weak.

I guess since I had been bed ridden for so long and then having the lung transplant surgery, it was considered normal to be so weak. Even though I worked so hard in rehab, I was told the strength it takes to get through a lung transplant and having been inactive for so long is major. Susan, the director of the rehab center had been an integral part of preparing me for the transplant. She was very calming and encouraging. Tuesday morning the nurse came in to change the dressing for my incision. She took the old dressing off and cleaned the incision. She said, "I don't even need to put a new dressing on the incision. It's already healed on the exterior. That's pretty amazing."

I was so happy. My family called me wonder woman. I sure didn't feel like wonder woman, but I guess considering what I had gone through it was pretty good. I noticed my frozen shoulder was gone. It must have been eliminated during surgery. All I know is frozen shoulder is very painful. It was completely gone. I was amazed by that.

Something else that was interesting is I was hallucinating in my hospital room. I never experienced that before. There were funny looking people (almost like a cross between a human and a ghost) looking at me from different places in the room—peaking around the window from outside, peaking from the crack in the bathroom door. They had looks on their faces like they were trying to spook me. I knew I was hallucinating and wasn't alarmed at all. I even said to them, "I know you are not real; don't think you are scaring me."

It was weird, I'll say that, but I knew it was hallucination. I told the nurse what I was experiencing, and we both thought it was due to the pain medication. I was probably on too big of a dose. She halved it and the problem went away.

Getting rid of the catheter was a milestone. Slowly but systematically the many tubes I had in me were removed except for the IV. I had tubes in my neck, my stomach, my right torso and my right arm. The rehab nurses were scheduled to start me walking on Wednesday, four days after surgery. We started very slowly. I used a walker. I could not believe how weak I was. It took immense core strength to walk to the bathroom from my bed, never mind walking on the hospital floor.

But I could breathe. No oxygen needed. I was in awe. I didn't eat or sleep for three days after my surgery. I remember the excited feeling I had. I knew it was a miracle. I didn't even think about what my condition was before the transplant. I just took on the new me. I could breathe. It was the best gift I could ever imagine.

One thing that was a little challenging was my brain needed to learn to work with my new right lung. My left lung was full of scleroderma and of little use. The brain needed to realize the left lung was no good and the right lung was perfect. It took a little while. I remember my breathing was short breathed and I couldn't take deep breaths or yawn. I was told the brain eventually figures it out to work with the good lung. Between the rehab and the breathing exercises after several weeks, my breathing was in synch and felt great. I knew it was a big milestone. The human body is truly amazing. I know exactly the moment when the brain figured it out. It was several days after I was home from the hospital. I have to say it was a little scary to not be able to take a deep breath until the brain and the new lung connected with each other. The nurses gave me confidence it would happen.

While still in the hospital, doctors came in to see me constantly and run tests. My eating was a little challenging with my esophagus problem. The GI specialist I saw before the transplant had said we'll watch you closely. You may need a feeding tube if worse comes to worse. I did not want a feeding tube. I did everything I could to avoid that one. I ate slowly. I didn't eat a lot. I remember the hospital food was so good though. I think in my mind I wanted to inhale it, but I knew my esophagus, and I didn't want to take any chances.

I was actually scheduled to go home after seven days. I thought it was too early by the way I felt. I ended up with an infection in my blood, and they kept me four more days. This type of infection wasn't that abnormal after a transplant. They had Center for Disease Control (CDC) doctors watching me. My energy healer, Mary, came to see me in the hospital too. She gave me an energy session to help with the healing. It was so comforting to see her. The nurses were all whispering, "What is she doing?" They were curious.

I was in the hospital for eleven days, and then home I went. What an effort that transition was, but I was determined. My mom and Nancy were with me visiting while in the hospital and after the hospital stay. The doctors and nurses at Inova Fairfax Hospital were amazing. I wasn't home very long. I had to go to the transplant clinic the day after I got home. They call it a post-transplant clinic visit at Inova Fairfax's Transplant Center. The transplant clinic visit consisted of chest x-ray, blood tests, breathing tests, and a visit with one of the pulmonologists in the group. They were all good.

My thought was why did they send me home if I had to turn around and go back the next day? I was cursing inside because it was such a physical effort. I was so weak. They wanted me to get use to the routine. No rest for the weary. The first week you go to the transplant clinic twice a week. The second week it's once a week. Then it's every other week and then once a month. You go to clinic once a month from that point on for the remainder of the first year after transplant. The first year you also go for a bronchoscopy every three months. You go to a pulmonary rehab center three times a week for the first six months with a lot of walking inside the house. You go to the transplant clinic every three months after the first year for the rest of your life.

It is indescribable how weak you are after the surgery. It was a busy time considering I was recovering from a major surgery. With so many transplant clinic trips and pulmonary rehab visits, it was craziness.

Thank you, Nancy and Mom for getting me through most of these visits. And thank you to all family and friends for the phone calls and cards and prayers. It helped me so much to get through the recovery process. I will remember your thoughtfulness always.

After a month of being home, I was able to get rid of the oxygen tank in my room. Even though I wasn't on oxygen any more, the doctors had wanted me to keep the oxygen tank for precautionary measures. It was a celebratory feeling to call the oxygen company and have them come pick it up and remove it from my house. It took a while for me to dare to light a candle even though I could have.

12

EMBRACE IT

The medications are a big deal. I was taking thirty-two pills per day at the beginning after transplant. There was a lot of drama on my part the first week. With the help and support of Nancy and my mom I got through it. I never took much medication my whole life. Taking pills of this magnitude was completely foreign to me. I accepted the fact that if I want to stay alive, I will be taking medications for the rest of my life; I better get used to it.

It's something you really have to manage. I have three different pills for antirejection. The antirejection medications are so you don't reject your organ. Then you have a lot of medications that are in response to side effects from the antirejection medications. As an example I developed high blood pressure from the antirejection medications and have to take blood pressure medication.

I developed a higher than normal creatinine level (kidney related) and am being monitored for that. There are antiviral and antibacterial medications you take because your immune system is seriously suppressed by the antirejection medications. Taking medications is part of your life, but I have to say, I am down to sixteen pills per day as my normal regimen. This is my daily cocktail to keep me alive for the rest of my life.

The antirejection pills you have to take every twelve hours as precisely as possible. Your rejection levels are checked every three months when you go for your transplant clinic visits. If the dose has to be adjusted based on your blood tests, you then go for a blood test after a week to see if the level is back to being in the range.

When you go for the blood test, the blood draw should be at the twelfth-hour mark before taking your next dose to get the true result. When you adjust the antirejection medication you automatically affect the creatinine level. If the creatinine level gets out of its range, you see a nephrologist, someone who specializes in the kidneys.

As the nephrologist said to me one visit, "Embrace it."

The only comments I'll make about the cocktail of medications I am on, are they make you very tired, and the tiredness is compounded by me having scleroderma symptoms as well. Fatigue and being abnormally cold are well-known symptoms with scleroderma patients. You are more susceptible to skin cancer from the medications so sun is not your friend.

My muscles were so atrophied after the surgery from being bed ridden and then going through the surgery and the medications also affect your muscle development, you have to work extra hard to bring you muscles back. Walking and exercise are very important. In some instances you've lost muscle so there is nothing to develop. It's a process. You do your best.

My mom and my sister were helpful and supported me through this process as well. I'd walk so slowly in a circle around my house from the living room to dining room to kitchen and back to living room. Maybe I started with two laps at a time and then improved as time went on. They would be cheering me on like I was doing a marathon. We would laugh about it. I would be so winded after those little walks.

I had to monitor my weight, blood pressure, temperature, and blood count (for diabetes) in the morning and before bed when I got home after my surgery. I had to keep a log and take it with me to the transplant clinic visits. This lasted the first six months basically.

It's really important to do what the doctors tell you to do. They know what they're doing.

During my recovery process, I developed severe stomach pain. I was hungry but I couldn't eat. I went to see my GI specialist who worked with the transplant team. Having a severe stomach issue with scleroderma and after this type of surgery and all the medications I was on, was not uncommon. I had been warned that there were added risks when doing a lung transplant on a scleroderma patient. I was doubled over in so much pain though, and I consider myself to have a high tolerance for pain. My mom and sister Nancy were by my side. I was in tears.

The GI specialist put me on a medication that worked miraculously after a few days, and the stomach problem went away totally in a couple of weeks. I was so relieved. I found myself thinking about what I wanted to eat in advance, like a whole day's worth. My mom and sister loved it because they didn't have to think about what to feed me.

When I really think about what is involved in being a caregiver, I realize it is not an easy job, especially for long periods of time. My mom and Nancy did a heroic job as they did the bulk of the care giving. It's scary when you have complications.

The weight gain was a slow process. I felt discouraged when I got on the scale to weigh myself: 100 pounds, then 98 pounds, then 100 pounds, then 99 pounds. After several weeks, my appetite finally took hold. It was kind of funny. Over time I went from size zero to a size two to a size four to a size six. It's hard to believe. When I was a size zero, I looked at the size six clothes I had and thought I'll never get in these clothes again. Look at how huge they are. I gave them to charity. Well, I'm there, a size six. Now I'm trying to lose a few pounds!

Around the fifth week after my transplant (October 2011), my cousin Sandy came to stay with me for a couple of weeks. My mom and Nancy were relieved to go home. Sandy and I had a fun visit. She decorated my outdoor entrance with fall flowers and pumpkins. I was in the process of getting a couple of shrubs replaced in the front of my house and was standing outside on the sidewalk watching the lawn contractor put the new shrubs in. I think Sandy saw I was struggling to stand and she came out and stood behind me with her hands around my waist. I was so thankful because I was trembling so much from weakness. It was going to take a good while to gain my strength back.

She took me to rehab visits, and she took me out for my first drive before she left to go back home. I was free at last. I could drive. I was a little shaky at first. After all, it had been almost a year since I drove.

Sandy actually stayed a little longer than anticipated. There was a major snow storm up north that took down power lines in some areas (hers was one of them). Schools were closed. It was a freak storm in October. The kids couldn't go trick or treating for Halloween because of the storm. We were fine in Maryland, no signs of stormy weather. She said "Why would I want to go home?" There is no electricity, lots of snow. She stayed right where she was for a few more days. I was happy to have her company. She's a great person.

Once I started driving on my own, I was able to go to the grocery store and doctor visits and rehab on my own. It was such a liberating feeling. I remember I went out to get yoga pants at a store. My wardrobe wasn't very exciting those days. I had a hard time standing and skimming through the racks at the store. I looked around and said OK no one is near me. I stooped down on one knee and looked up at the pants. It was easier to stoop down and look up than to stand up. You do what you've got to do. But I was determined to get strong again.

Another complication I had. My bone marrow was abnormal; specifically my white blood cell count was low. I had to give myself Neupogen shots to try to bring the white blood cell count up. There was a little drama with this. The doctors expected me to give myself the shots. They were prefilled with the prescription.

It was a big needle, humongous. I couldn't do it. I begged the director of the rehab center to give me the shot. She is a nurse. She was such a good sport about it. Sometimes she had a backup in her absence. I think I had to have the shot twice a week for a few weeks.

I went for a bone marrow biopsy to rule out cancer. They have to scrape your bone to get a sample for testing. It hurt like hell. Thankfully, there was no cancer. The bone doctor advised that I could get off the Neupogen shots. The blood test results were acceptable considering the medications I was on.

Thank you, God. I can't say enough about all the doctors I had. They just knew what to do always. I was so dependent on them.

Rehab continued for six months after my transplant. Then you are on your own to exercise. There was a community center right down the street from my house that had an exercise room with equipment. It was perfect. That's where I planned to go after my six months were up.

Sue came to visit me for Thanksgiving. It was comforting. She even decorated a tabletop metal Christmas tree with my most prized decorations that I love. At my three month mark I went to Connecticut for Christmas 2011 by train. The trip to Connecticut took a lot out of me, but it was therapeutic to do this on my own and see my family. We had a big

Christmas bash as usual. I also saw my friend JoAnn, and I went to a party at her brother's house. It was a great feeling to be experiencing life again. I was fragile but I put on a brave face. I had confidence I would get stronger and stronger. I was happy and proud of myself.

For one of my transplant clinic visits, my scheduled doctor was called out on an emergency so I got to see the director of the clinic, Dr. Nathan. I was telling him how thankful I am for this miracle of a lung transplant. I was going on and on about how I was before and how I am after. He asked me if he could interview me. He liked my enthusiasm. I said, "You mean now?"

He said, "Yes." So he proceeded to get his laptop and we went through the interview. It was a short one, probably fifteen minutes long. He said he would use it in his training classes. He showed it to me. It was pretty good for being impromptu.

It seemed like every three months I hit a milestone of gaining strength. I was encouraged.

The first year was the toughest. You have to be careful what you eat. Your body is healing internally, so as an example, I didn't want to develop diabetes which is common after a transplant caused by the antirejection medications you are taking. I stayed away from sugar completely for at least six months. Vegetables and Fruit had to be peeled and cooked, which we probably did for the first six months. Then I started to ease into raw vegetables and fruit, still peeled, an apple, for example. I had to be selective about where I would eat out too. It's the immunosuppressant drugs I have to be on that make me susceptible. Thankfully, I have not developed any infections or sickness so far. I believe being careful what you eat helped a lot and still does.

Muscle weakness is another important aspect. As hard as it was, I had to exercise as much as possible to build up the atrophied muscle. Having been bedridden for the most part of a year didn't help the situation even with the rehabilitation exercise and the many doctor visits. It took every bit of energy I had to gain strength back and be independent.

The antirejection medications slow down your muscle development. Therefore, gaining physical strength back is a work in progress. Having the type of scleroderma that I have makes the process a bit challenging because you have a whole set of scleroderma symptoms with which you deal on a daily basis.

Miraculously the new lung allows you to breathe again. And the scleroderma will not return in the new lung because the new lung has a different cell make-up. Isn't that interesting? The connective tissue, though, is produced in other parts of your body and causes adverse symptoms, for example, calcium deposits, Raynaud's (always cold no matter how warmly you dress), GI challenges (digestive system), tightness in the face and hands, muscle weakness, fatigue, broken blood vessels on hands and face. I referenced earlier, the symptoms are more of a nuisance, not life threatening, but they can really wear you out.

The effects from the cocktail of medications I am on compounds the situation. I am often shaky. Scleroderma can be deceiving because you can appear to look good but internally not so good. You become selective on how you use your energy, and you have good days and bad days from an energy perspective. I have to say I have accepted my condition and have learned how to live with it.

I've learned my limitations, and I know when I can push myself. I don't consider myself a victim. I am a victor. Every day of life is a gift beyond belief. And I live it to the best of my ability. So much of life is a state of mind. I remember hearing a speaker say that what counts is how you deal with your medical challenges while you are alive. It takes strength and courage. I agree.

Breathing is a beautiful thing.

It was April 2012. There was an annual celebration event in the District of Columbia sponsored by Washington Regional Transplant Center (WRTC). This event was for organ recipients and organ donor families to get together and celebrate. I was in my eighth month after lung transplant.

It was a very moving and emotional event for everyone who attended. There were guest speakers and remembrances of those who passed away and donated their organ. There were donor recipients who were at all different stages. It seemed like there were close to 500 people in attendance. It was my first time going to this annual event. My sister Pat and my neighbor Jackie went with me. My sister took the train down from Connecticut to Maryland to be with me.

What impressed me the most about this event is that donor families could see how much a donated organ positively impacts others, and it also was an eye opening experience for the recipients to see the impact on the donor families for their loss of life. No one knows who they are matched up with unless both parties previously agreed to meet after the transplant through the WRTC.

I was sitting next to a family who had lost their one-year-old baby. They were holding a square patch made out of fabric and included a picture of their little girl. I decided to ask them about their little girl. They were so happy to talk about her. They donated the baby's organs which was amazing to me. There are many young children who need organs. There was a quilt that was going to be memorialized during the event and a video of all recent donors who had passed away and whose families had donor patches to add to the quilt. I was touched and teary eyed.

So the event went on. There were two guest speakers who were transplant recipients. The first one underwent a heart transplant as an infant and years later went on to become a heart doctor. That was very inspiring. The other speaker had been severely burned in a fire and received several skin transplants. Both were significant life-saving events.

Then there was the quilt memoriam. Each donor family walked up individually and presented their donor patch for incorporation onto the quilt. Once that quilt was at its right size the WRTC would go on to start another quilt. I think there were four large quilts hanging on the wall that had already been completed.

Then came the celebration of life honoring recipients. The speaker said a few words about the gift of organ donation and asked for those recipients that were twenty-five years or more to stand up and stay standing. There actually was one person who stood up. I was shocked. They went on to ask for those between fifteen and twenty-five years; a few more stood up. Then those between five and fifteen years and then those under five years (that's when I stood up). We were all standing, and they also asked for the recipient's family members to stand up. It was uplifting to see everyone who was standing, all walks of life, different cultures, and different ages.

When I stood up the family next to me whose baby girl was a donor looked up at me in surprise and smiled. They had no idea I was a recipient. They asked what kind of transplant I had, and I told them lung. We all hugged. It was a poignant moment because we both had experienced the other side of the organ donation experience.

The final portion of the event was moving too. Facilitators went to each row and gave out lit candles one by one to pass down the row so that everyone in the large room had a lit candle. A professional sang a beautiful song and then we all blew out our candle. I was so glad I went to the event and to have my sister and my neighbor with me was special.

Something else that was very special, my visit with the operating nurse, Ann Marie, who helped me off the ventilator. It was several months after my surgery. I wanted to thank her and show her how I was doing. I called ahead of time to coordinate the visit as I know how busy she is. It was so lucky.

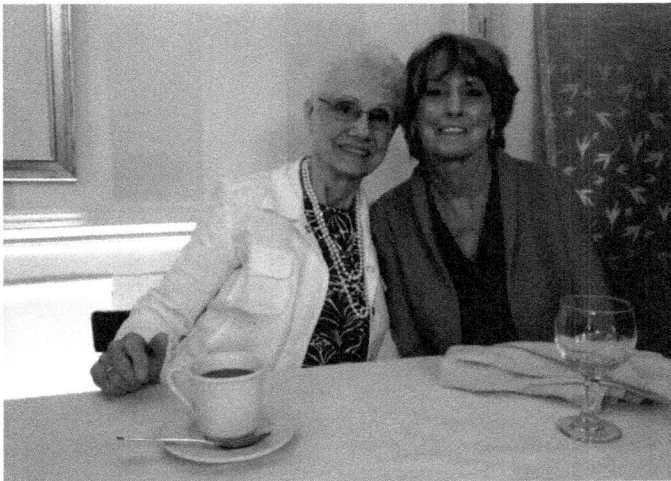

Figure 2. Eight months post-surgery with Mom

We spent a good half hour together. I brought a card with a thoughtful note. We shared tears together. She was really touched. She said she had never seen a patient after they left the hospital. To see a patient breathing and functioning was very rewarding she said. She thanked me and I thanked her and we hugged. It was such a good feeling.

13

NEVER GIVE UP

In May 2012, I went to Connecticut to see my mother on Mother's day. In July 2012, I flew to New Hampshire to see my brother and his family. We went up to Maine one day to see my cousin Sandy who had graciously taken time out of her life to take care of me in October 2011 after my transplant. She has a winterized cottage near the water. It was fun visiting Maine and New Hampshire. After all, I lived in that area for twenty-two years. I remember feeling very tired, but I wanted to show that I was doing well.

I went to Connecticut for Thanksgiving and Christmas 2012 to see family. I went by train. There was a little excitement this Connecticut trip. On Thanksgiving I had a terrible backache. I thought I slept wrong the night before. My sister Sue noticed a bulge on my neck and didn't like that. I hadn't noticed it. But she also thought I might be getting Shingles and that's why my back ached. Well it turned out I was getting shingles. Once it was confirmed, I called the transplant clinic and they called in a prescription to a local Pharmacy as well as something for the pain. Shingles was pretty painful. It landed on my body right in the area of my lung transplant surgery. The pain lasted for several weeks.

My mom, my sister Nancy and her husband Joe (visiting Mom from Florida) had gone out for dinner one night and brought me back some pizza. I was sitting at the kitchen table eating the pizza, and I started to feel dizzy. I decided to walk to the bathroom not too far away. That was a mistake. I passed out in the bathroom bruising my entire face. It was a small powder room so I must have hit everything. My brother-in-law Joe talked to me on the floor to try and bring me back to consciousness again. It was only a matter of seconds before I became conscious, but I couldn't figure out why I was on the floor. My face was swelling up. I could feel it as I lay on my back. My sister Nancy called the ambulance, and they proceeded to take me to St. Raphael's Hospital in New Haven, Connecticut. The hospital staff had a CT scan done of the head which showed no problems thank goodness. I was kept overnight for observation. They said my blood count was a little low but I was discharged the next day.

My brother Tom picked me up and took me home. He was shocked at how bruised my face was. Before we left I was wheeled down to the first floor to get my transplant medications which the hospital wouldn't let me take while I was in the hospital. The hospital staff was required to provide any medications from their own pharmacy. The entire trip in the wheel chair people would look at me strangely. I really looked like I was beat up. My brother candidly responded with his hands up, I didn't do it! The nurse and I had a good laugh.

Christmas Eve I was supposed to go to my sister Sue's house. She's had Christmas Eve at her house for years. I didn't go. I had too much going on. My mom brought me back some Christmas Eve dinner. I was so tired. Christmas was OK. I went to my sister Pat's looking like a freak with my face all bruised.

No photos that Christmas. A couple of days after Christmas I was unusually tired. I tested my oxygen when I went to bed. It was very low. I stayed awake all night. I felt I needed to go to the hospital. I thought I might be rejecting my organ. It was the first scare I had (and the last so far). I was going to call an ambulance, but at six o'clock in the morning, I called my brother Tom to let him know what I was doing, and he offered to pick me up at my mom's house and take me to Yale-New Haven Hospital.

My brother urgently told the hospital personnel at the emergency room that I am a post lung transplant patient. No questions were asked. I was admitted on the spot. The weather prediction was snow storm. I must have had the best room in the hospital. I think I have my brother to thank for that. When I looked out my window the snow was really coming down. I told my brother he should leave. The weather is not good. I was so appreciative he got me to the hospital.

The hospital staff had to rule out certain conditions with several tests to try to come to a conclusion as to why my oxygen level was so low. All the tests showed my lung was fine. The prognosis was I was severely anemic. It turned out dapsone, one of the medications I was on for only a month at this point, can cause severe anemia. Ever since my transplant, I had been receiving an injection of a medication that took about a half hour once a month at the hospital as an outpatient procedure to prevent PCP pneumonia, but there became a shortage of this medication so they put me on a medication called dapsone.

You have to have a test before you start taking dapsone to see if your body can tolerate it, mainly your red blood cell count. I passed the test so I started taking it in November 2012. Nearly a month later I had to have a blood transfusion. I learned there are several types of blood transfusions. Mine was a plasma only transfusion. It straightened me out. The hospital staff kept me for two nights, and I begged them to let me go so I could celebrate New Year's Eve and most of all start off the New Year with a clean slate from any medical mishaps. They agreed.

Needless to say, they took me off the dapsone. I never got on a different medicine for this specific pneumonia. It wasn't a common pneumonia, but if you do get it, it's severe and difficult to eradicate. I consulted with my scleroderma specialist at that time and decided on my own it was not a big risk to not be treated for this PCP pneumonia. I would take my chances. Back to Maryland I went January 14. It was a much longer stay than I had anticipated.

One other situation I had to address. I needed to find out why I had that bulge on my neck. I did have a lot of veins on my chest that protruded mostly on the left side of my chest opposite from where my lung transplant surgery was. My take was the doctors had to move the veins over to get the lung inside. I'm so smart aren't I? I finally did remember to ask the doctors about the bulge on my neck at the next transplant clinic appointment. They didn't like it and sent me immediately to have an ultrasound.

The results revealed I had three small blood clots in my neck most likely from the surgery. I would need to be on Coumadin. The doctors anticipated me being on the Coumadin for six months. I prayed six months would do the trick as there was a special diet you had to follow and get your blood tested often to see that the blood levels were within a certain range. It all worked out. The clots went away for the most part and the doctors attribute the protruded veins in my chest to be a "war wound" from my surgery. They wouldn't go away but thankfully my body had found other routes for the blood to flow in my chest.

As the doctors would tell me from time to time, "Embrace it".

14

THE MIRACLE IS AN AMAZING PROCESS

I never lose sight of my previous life, and all the greatness about it. I had so many life experiences and fulfilling times, very fast paced, many challenging and personal growth opportunities. What I like about it is I shared most of it with others. I have many good memories to make me smile for the rest of my life. When one door closes, another door opens (another Spanish proverb). Now I am able to enjoy the simple things in life much more...love, family, friends, nature, giving back. Not so attached to material things. I try to keep stress out of my life as much as I can. I understand faith, hope and charity so much more now. Love of friends and family and my faith in God are what got me through and continue to keep me going.

In retrospect, as positive and hopeful as I was, dealing with my illness, I realize now more than ever how close I was to dying. The lung transplant saved my life. I would not be alive to tell this story if I didn't receive the transplant when I did. When we found out Inova Fairfax was willing to do the transplant despite the fact that I have scleroderma with advanced lung disease caused by scleroderma, so much still had to happen. I still had to go through the extensive qualification process to get on the list, and then I had to maintain my health standing and also wait for a matching lung. I only had so much time. As some people said, I looked like I was ninety years old. I was so thin and aged. Well the transplant really did save my life. It was a miracle. Now I can breathe and live my life to the fullest possible. I have scleroderma which is no picnic but I can breathe! You basically can't do anything without the ability to breathe. Life is a precious gift now that I have it back again.

In February 2013 after the escapades in Connecticut, I thought maybe I should think about being closer to my family. This was after my brother Tom encouraged me to move to Connecticut. I had been in Maryland for fourteen years, which includes the two years after my transplant. I didn't have any family in Maryland, and I didn't want to put my family through having to travel back and forth, God forbid anything happened to me. I talked with family members about selling my house in Maryland and moving up North. It was interesting; I never lived close geographically to my family my whole adult life. It would be different.

A lot of things entered my mind. I had to think about a change in doctors (I was very attached to my doctors). I had to find a good sales agent to help me sell my house in Maryland. I had to find a place to live in Connecticut. How was I going to do it all? Initially, I thought I wasn't ready to leave my home and friends. It was too overwhelming. But then something came over me and I said I have to do this now. If I wait, it won't get any easier. Maybe it was Rebecca guiding me? I don't know. The decision came on me pretty quickly.

I began reflecting on the adjustment I've been making from being employed and thriving with a thirty-five-year career to reaching a point where I had to leave work for serious health reasons. I wanted to do something to give back for the gift I received. I really wanted to help pre-lung transplant patients by mentoring them for pre- and post-transplant. I became an ambassador for the Donate Life Organization in Maryland. I went through the training and attended many of the events where I had an opportunity to share my transplant experience. I would bump into pre-transplant patients at my transplant clinic visits and talk with them about the transplant experience. They were eager to hear about it, and I was happy to enlighten them with the good experience I had. I was on the Inova Fairfax Hospital's list in Virginia where I had my transplant to speak at their Information Days for pre-transplant patients.

I was enjoying my independence, free from oxygen, getting involved with community again and socializing with friends. I had my limitations but I was living life, taking care of myself, and volunteering. That made me happy. I knew when I needed to rest.

Meanwhile, I was on a mission to get to Connecticut; onward and upward. No pun intended. There was so much to do. I informed my friends in Maryland of my decision. I could count my close friends on one hand but they were great. They supported me as they always did. I cherish them and the life experience we shared from knowing each other. We still keep in touch. It was sad in some ways, but we all knew it was the right thing for me to do. I informed my doctors. The lung transplant center director at Inova Fairfax Hospital in Virginia personally knows the lung transplant center director at New York Presbyterian Hospital in New York City and immediately began making arrangements for the transfer. There is no lung transplant center in Connecticut.

My scleroderma specialist at Johns Hopkins Scleroderma Center supported my decision as well. It wasn't going to be easy leaving her. Scleroderma people travel from all over the country to the scleroderma center at Johns Hopkins. There is only one scleroderma specialist in Connecticut, who practices at the University of Connecticut, which isn't very close to where my family lives. I would figure something out. I also had to find a GI specialist and a kidney specialist. These were my main doctors in addition to the Lung Transplant Center. I resigned from the board of the townhouse association in which I lived. I had stepped down from being president after I left work and went on disability (in June 2010) but had remained on the board as a member at large mainly as a resource.

I called my bank and asked my contact in the mortgage department if she had dealt with a good sales agent who was better than the rest. I have to say I could not have been given a better sales agent. He was the cream of the crop. Not your average sales agent for sure. He wasn't just out for the sale. Call it luck of the draw. I say the stars were aligned. I really needed him because I was in a semi-weakened state. It was eighteen months after my transplant and I was downsizing my home tremendously knowing I would be moving into a much smaller place. I used every charity known to man. My neighbors even took a few large items. My house was put on the market in May 2013. It sold in four days; closing on June 28. What a whirlwind.

There was a condo in Connecticut that I was looking to get through my sister-in-law's stepmother. It wouldn't be available until the fall, so I would live with my mom until I could move. All of my personal items would be put in storage. I was so exhausted when I got to Connecticut at my mom's it was an understatement. I don't know how I did the move on my own. Well I know what it was. It was adrenaline that made it happen. My adrenaline was still available to tap into. I've found throughout my life when something needs to happen you just do it. The adrenaline kicks in and you handle it.

I think in a lot of cases being the oldest in a family has some influence too. Or maybe it's as simple as being in survival mode. Whatever it is, I always strived to make the best of it and get the most out of it that I can, accentuating the positive and eliminating the negative. It's the story of my life. My friend JoAnn came down to Maryland on the train and drove to Connecticut with me after the closing on my house. I even drove the whole way. It went by fast. We had a good time catching up and having some laughs. I couldn't believe I was making this major transition. I did it. June 29, 2013.

I called a woman I was friends with in high school, Carol, to let her know I was now in Connecticut. I had been in touch with her when I lived in Maryland because my mom ran into her up in Connecticut and told her about my condition. She coordinated a dinner with a small group of us who hung out together in high school (Carol, Judy, Melissa, JoAnn, Eileen). It was really a lot of fun. One of the women, Judy, lives in Oklahoma but was visiting so it was great. Another is a nurse at Yale New Haven Hospital, Eileen. Eileen offered to help me with finding doctors. Talk about no coincidences. She connected me with the best GI specialist who knew all the right doctors for me. I'm happy with all of them. Remember I said earlier there is no scleroderma specialist in Connecticut except one at the University of Connecticut (UConn), which is far from where I was living. The rheumatologist I was given by the GI doctor attended UConn and was trained by the scleroderma specialist at UConn. She is very familiar with scleroderma. I like her so much. This was a great find since in Maryland I was seeing a scleroderma specialist at Johns Hopkins Scleroderma Center; the best of the best.

After being at my mom's for a couple of months, I decided I wanted to look into volunteering in some capacity. I called the library in the town where I would be living once I purchased my condo. The library didn't have a need for any more volunteers but they suggested I call a specific charity in the town.

The timing couldn't have been more perfect. They were in need of someone on Mondays and Fridays. I signed up and started right away. The drive was about fifteen minutes away from my mom's house. When I moved into my condo in January 2014, I had a seven-minute commute; a far cry from the commutes I had when I lived in the Maryland, DC, Virginia area. So much change. But for the most part I go with the flow. Everything happens for a reason. I've been enjoying the volunteer job a lot. I feel part of the team. I need that. And it feels good to give back. Helping others helps keep the focus off me and my condition.

I moved into my condo January 31, 2014; a condo different than I had originally planned on. Luckily another condo unit opened up in the same complex. I think it was divine intervention. The timing was impeccable. I grabbed it. The woman who owned the original condo I was interested in decided she wasn't ready to move. Given her situation I could understand that. She is an older woman and very independent.

My sister Sue and her daughter Katie were phenomenal with the move. They took charge of unpacking everything and putting everything in its place for me. I helped as much as I could. It was unbelievable that they took the reins and did a beautiful job. It was a big undertaking. Coming from Maryland, I wasn't adjusted to the New England winters at all. I'm still waiting for the adjustment to happen! Heritage Sound is the name of the association in Milford where I live, a shoreline town. I live a couple of minutes away from the water and there is a new boardwalk that connects one beach to another. The town of Milford is charming. It's a great little town for my new life. I'm very happy with my new surroundings. I live close enough to family members which makes me feel safe. My family is the best. I really appreciate them. I do everything I can to take care of myself independently. My brother Tom does take me to the lung transplant center in New York City every three months. It's our bonding time. I'm so grateful for this. It's one of those things you don't want to have to do by yourself.

I feel very fortunate I have been given the gift of life, a second chance. It's the miracle I so desperately needed. I have embraced my new life. I am living life and going at my own pace. I am a solid seven on a scale of one to ten. And I hope to even get better. Considering I was a one before the transplant, a seven is remarkable. I take care of myself, my condo, food shop, walk, go to a movie, go out to dinner, handle my personal business, volunteer, and other events. I manage my medications and doctor appointments.

One day my friend JoAnn and I went shelling at the beach something I hadn't done since I was sick. On the way home, it dawned on me I was singing a song playing on the radio. I couldn't sing before. Not enough lung capacity. It was such a happy feeling. I belted the song out. I have been to a club and danced, and I've even enjoyed a concert on the green singing and dancing in front of the stage (Billy Joel Tribute Band). These things you take for granted until you can't do them. It brings tears to my eyes. I haven't gone under the water yet. I'll get there. I rest when I need to in between activities.

My new scleroderma specialist who I am thrilled to know connected me with a patient who has scleroderma and is considering a lung transplant. The doctor asked if I would talk with this patient about my lung transplant experience. I said of course. I am so very happy to share my experiences. I really want to do more of this. Helping others learn about what to expect is something I did in Maryland when there was an opportunity and loved it. We'll see what else the universe has in store for me. I'm game. Whatever happens, my perspective is that the journey is the reward. You want to make the best of everything in life. I've learned there are a few other scleroderma patients in the area. There aren't many of us around. We're going to try to connect and support each other.

There is always someone who is dealing with something worse. Everybody has something. For me, coping with my chronic illness involves having faith in God, thinking positive and dealing with it head on. The love of friends and family also plays an integral part. Experiencing love means a lot. It's such a give and take. It's a beautiful thing just like breathing is. You have to be positive to keep yourself strong. Ultimately, you are your own best advocate.

www.ingramcontent.com/pod-product-compliance
Lightning Source LLC
LaVergne TN
LVHW051840080426
835512LV00018B/2987